Healthy Echoes

f.h

A Mother's Influence on Health

A 3-Month Mother-Daughter Health Journey

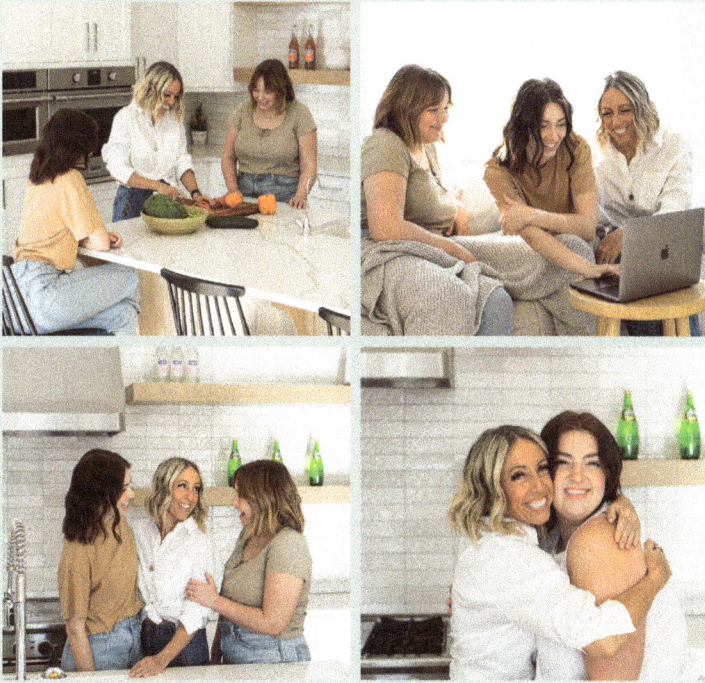

Healthy Echoes is more than a weight loss program. It is a life-changing experience designed to inspire a positive view of body image and a healthier relationship with food, nurturing a legacy of self-confidence and well-being for both mothers and daughters. Learn about preventing PCOS, diabetes, and the role of muscle in insulin resistance, and sustainable weight management. I am excited to present this empowering journey toward healthier, happier relationships with your bodies, your food, and each other.

created by
func. health with Maggie Topham

Healthy Echoes

Introduction

Welcome to our Wellness Course, a transformative journey designed exclusively for mothers and daughters to embark on together. We believe in fostering a strong, positive relationship with your bodies and food because health goes beyond numbers on a scale. It is about embracing wellness as a lifestyle, where self-love, self-care, and disease prevention become our guiding principles.

In a world that often bombards us with unrealistic beauty standards and quick-fix diets, we empower you with the tools and knowledge to create a sustainable, nurturing, and loving relationship with your bodies.

We understand that the mother-daughter bond is unique and powerful, and it provides the perfect foundation for inspiring change and mutual support. Our program is not about deprivation or unrealistic expectations. It is about understanding your bodies, nourishing them, and growing together in health and self-confidence.

This course will guide you on a journey toward wellness through this educational resource. As you embark on this empowering path, you will learn to appreciate your bodies for the incredible vessels they are and develop a healthier relationship with food. With a focus on self-acceptance, gaining knowledge, and confidence in health choices, you and your daughter will transform physically, emotionally, and mentally.

created by
func. health with Maggie Topham

Healthy Echoes

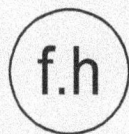

Instructions

Throughout this mother-daughter course, we are excited to introduce a rhythm that is both fun and easy to follow! Every two weeks, we will unwrap a brand-new module during our 3-month course. And guess what? Each one has its own awesome elements:

- **Time to Learn**: Every module will begin with a "Let's Learn" segment that delves into essential topics related to your well-being, such as body image, label reading, nutrition, emotional eating, rest, and exercise.

- **Ready, Set, Goal**: You and your daughter will team up to set a goal for the module. Think of it as your superpower challenge! Something to work on together, one step at a time.

- **Identify Roadblocks**: You will encounter difficult moments as you evolve with your new lifestyle changes. We call these moments roadblocks. By writing them down, you acknowledge them and then can move forward with purpose.

- **Pen to Paper:** Prepare your pencils because we have worksheets! These are like our secret weapons for making these ideas stick. They will help you apply what you have learned, evaluate your understanding, and have some fun along the way.

- **Accountability CTA (Call to Action)**: At the conclusion of each module, you will both be encouraged to participate in an Accountability CTA. This will involve discussing your experiences, challenges, and successes with each other while offering and receiving support and maintaining your commitment to each other and your progress.

Get ready to roll on this empowering adventure. I am thrilled to be a part of your journey, and I cannot wait for you to see the sustainable changes you and your daughter will make together as she echoes your desire to love and care for her body!

created by
func. health with Maggie Topham

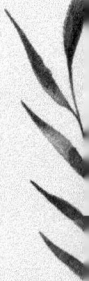

Body Image & Nutrition

Eating well is the first act of love for your body

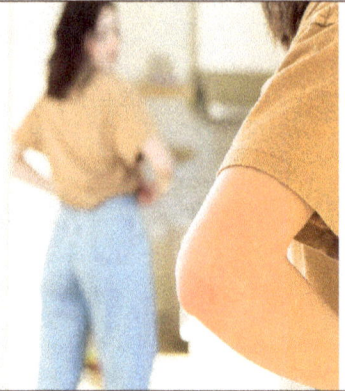

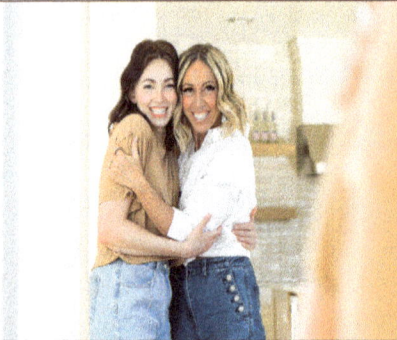

Welcome to Module #1! We are excited that you are taking this journey together as a mother and daughter. This unique partnership between mothers and daughters can have a profound impact on body image, body love, and self-confidence.

Topics in this Module

- Modeling behavior
- Eliminating sugar - crowd it out
- Nutrition brings confidence
- Shared experiences & growth

In this Module, we will delve into the science behind the mother-daughter relationship and its role in shaping our perception of our bodies. We will also explore the importance of healthy eating, and crowding out sugar. Most importantly, we will approach the benefits of embracing and appreciating our bodies.

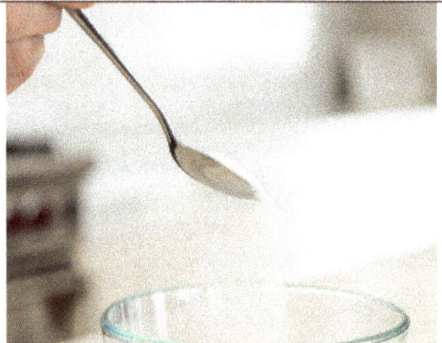

Notes _____

_____

_____

Time to Learn

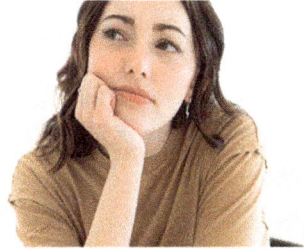

Page 1

The Mother-Daughter Relationship and Body Image

The mother-daughter relationship is a powerful force in shaping how we perceive our bodies. Studies have shown that mothers significantly influence their daughters' body image, positively or negatively. Your interactions, conversations, and attitudes toward your body are a mirror for your daughter. Here is how your relationship can impact body image and body love:

1. **Modeling Behavior:** Your daughter learns from your behavior. If she sees you embracing and loving your body, she is more likely to do the same. If you criticize your own body, she may internalize similar self-criticism.

2. **Communication:** Open and honest conversations about body image and self-esteem are essential. Encourage each other to share your feelings, concerns, and insecurities, and respond with empathy and support.

3. **Shared Experiences**: Exercising together, cooking healthy meals as a team, or sharing recipes via text and participating in wellness activities can be bonding experiences that foster positive body image and build confidence.

Notes _____

_____

_____

Time to Learn

The Importance of Healthy Eating

Let's talk about healthy eating. Nutrition plays a vital role in how we feel about our bodies and ourselves. Cutting out sugar can be a significant step toward better health and wellness. Here is why it is important:

1. **The Impact Sugar has on the Body**: Excess sugar consumption can lead to weight gain, skin problems, energy spikes and crashes, and even mood swings. It is not just about calories; it is also about the effect sugar has on our bodies.

2. **Reducing Sugar Improves Health**: Cutting out or at least reducing added sugars in your diet can lead to better blood sugar control, lower risk of chronic diseases like type 2 diabetes and heart disease, and improved overall health. Reducing sugar leaves room for nutrient-dense foods.

3. **Mental Health**: Your diet can affect your mental health. Excessive sugar intake has been linked to an increased risk of depression and anxiety. By choosing healthier options, you can support both your physical and mental well-being.

Notes _____

Time to Learn

Steps to Crowd out Sugar

Here are three steps to help you crowd out sugar (move it aside as you replace it with something nutritious) or eliminate it from your diet:

1. **Read Labels**: Start by reading food labels. Look for hidden sources of sugar like high fructose corn syrup, sucrose, and other sweeteners. Be mindful of processed foods and sugary drinks.

2. **Opt for Natural Sweeteners**: When you need a sweet fix, choose natural alternatives like honey or maple syrup in moderation. Fresh fruits can also satisfy your sweet tooth without the harmful effects of added sugar.

3. **Meal Planning**: Plan your meals together and include whole, unprocessed foods; prioritize protein and include whole foods high in fiber with healthy fats to help eliminate sugar cravings and encourage a stronger feeling of satiety (feeling satisfied or full).

Embracing and Appreciating Our Bodies

The ultimate goal in your health and wellness journey is to build self-confidence and appreciate your bodies for what they are. This practice can help combat the negative influence of social media and unrealistic expectations. Here's how:

1. **Boosted Confidence**: When you embrace your bodies and practice self-love, it boosts your self-esteem and confidence. You become less susceptible to the unrealistic beauty standards presented on social media.

Notes

Time to Learn

2. **Resilience**: Accepting and appreciating your bodies makes you more resilient to criticism. You'll learn to value what truly matters – your health, happiness, and self-worth – over fleeting external ideals.

3. **Positive Influence**: By cultivating body love and self-confidence together, you positively influence each other. You can counteract the toxic influences of social media and unrealistic expectations by showing that happiness and well-being are more important than appearance.

Remember, this journey is about health and wellness, not perfection. Your bond as a mother and daughter is a powerful tool in nurturing a positive body image and building self-confidence. Encourage each other, communicate openly, and share the triumphs and setbacks along the way. You are not alone in this – you have each other's support and love, and that's a beautiful foundation for a healthier and happier life.

Embracing a healthier lifestyle, cutting out excess sugar, and cultivating body love will empower each of you to navigate the complexities of social media and its impact on body image with grace and resilience. As you embark on this journey together, remember that every small step towards a healthier, happier life is a significant achievement. Your health and happiness are worth it, and your bond as mother and daughter is a great strength as you show accountability and support to each other. You are a whole step closer to your goals today than you were yesterday!

Notes ⎯⎯⎯⎯⎯⎯⎯⎯⎯⎯⎯⎯⎯⎯⎯⎯⎯⎯⎯⎯⎯⎯⎯⎯⎯⎯⎯⎯⎯⎯⎯

Pen to Paper

It's time to go to work!

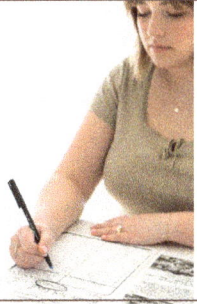

Page 5

Daughter's Worksheet

How have you felt about your mom's self-body image and dialogue? Do you think it has affected your perception of your body or self-worth in any way?

Have you ever felt pressured to meet certain beauty standards because of something your mom said or did? How could you help her to understand?

Is there anything specific about your mom's relationship with her body or food that you'd like to talk about or feel has influenced your own choices?

What's your experience with social media and body image? Do you ever feel influenced by the images or messages you see online?"

Do you ever find yourself using the same wording or phrases your mom uses about her body? If so, write them down and talk about it together.

Notes

Pen to Paper

It's time to go to work!

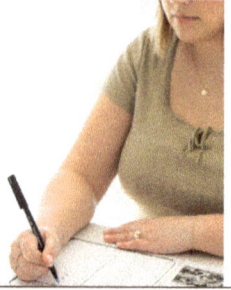

Page 6

Mom's Worksheet

How do you handle the influence of social media on your own body image and self-esteem? Do you have any strategies to help your daughter deal with it?

Have you ever experienced peer pressure or societal expectations about your body that you think might have influenced your relationship with food or your body?

What has been your journey towards body acceptance, and do you have any tips for your daughter to navigate this path?

How have you approached teaching your daughter about her body image in the past? How would you like to improve?

How can we, as a mother-daughter team, work together to promote a positive self-body image and navigate the challenges of social media in a healthy way?

Notes _____

_____

_____

Ready, Set, Goal!

It's time for some self-reflection & goal-setting!

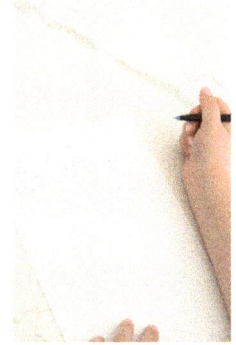

Page 7

Worksheet Wrap-up

These questions are designed to foster open and constructive conversations between mothers and daughters. We hope to encourage enlightenment and understanding about the influence of self-body image, dialogue, and external factors on your wellness and self-confidence. Remember, the key is to create a safe and non-judgmental space for these discussions, where both of you, as mother and daughter, can share your thoughts, feelings, and experiences.

Learning the importance of modeling behavior has shined some light on your words and attitudes toward your bodies. The conversations you shared together through the previous worksheet will be the beginning of a mindset change. The mind is our most powerful tool! The love and appreciation you show for your body starts there.

Your body has gotten you this far! It is probably time to thank her for her hard work. The best act of appreciation is by nurturing your body with the proper fuel to encourage healthy muscle and lowered fat stores. This is called metabolic health. As you work on your metabolic health, you will be surprised by your boost in confidence. Just knowing you're doing something positive for your body is powerful, especially as you support and report to each other.

The following exercise is to help you set a Module #1 goal together. Remember, this is not about deprivation; it is about making wise nutritional choices that encourage replacing a poor choice with a smarter choice.

Notes _____

_____

_____

Ready, Set, Goal!

Crowd Out Sugar!

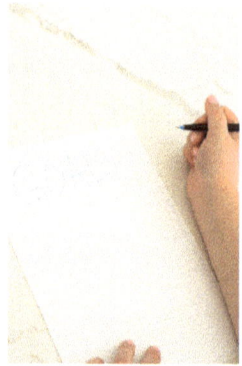

Page 8

This model includes a goal sheet that will require daily reflection and a record of your experience surrounding body image and nutrition. Keep the following information in mind when meeting these goals.

You'll be asked to "crowd out sugar." Here is why:

Sugar consumption leads to higher glucose levels. Higher glucose levels lead to higher insulin levels. Higher insulin levels lock up fat and force your body to only burn sugar. Whether you are on this journey to lose weight or just improve your health, your body needs the flexibility to use both body fat AND sugar as fuel. This is called metabolic flexibility, and it is something you want! Using body fat for fuel (ketones) instead of sugar (glucose) leads to fewer energy crashes, cravings, and mood swings. It also promotes a healthy body weight and the shedding of extra body fat. These body conditions also help fight diseases like PCOS, obesity, diabetes, heart disease, and Alzheimer's. Are you convinced yet?!

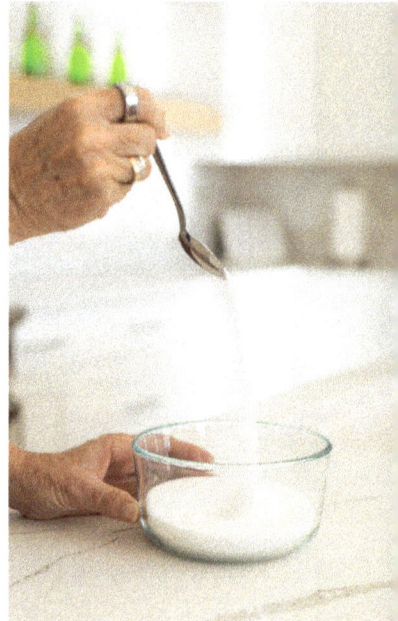

Notes

Ready, Set, Goal!

Show that body some LOVE!

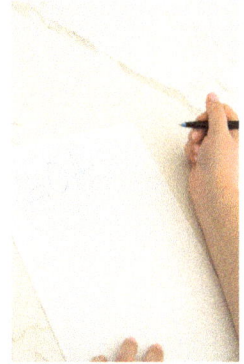

Page 9

Changing your mindset to embrace body love involves shifting your focus from self-criticism to self-acceptance. Recognize that your body is unique and has carried you through life's journey. Value its strength and resilience. We can celebrate the beauty that comes from self-confidence and self-compassion. Accept that your body is a gift and the only one you have got!

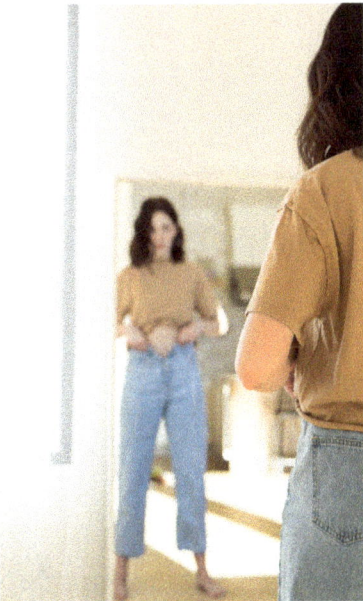

You will be asked to appreciate your body. Here is why:

Daily body affirmations, combined with healthy food choices, have a profound impact on your mindset. Affirmations promote self-love and acceptance, fostering a positive body image. When you nourish your body with healthy foods, you signal self-care and respect, reinforcing self-worth. This positive reinforcement boosts confidence and changes your mindset from one of criticism to one that values and appreciates your body. This leads to a happier and healthier relationship with yourself and the perfect defense against outside influences and old beliefs. Perfection is NOT health. Your individual characteristics are what is beautiful about you!

Notes

Ready, Set, Goal!

Page 10   (For Mom)

Show that body some LOVE by crowding out sugar!

Write down one thing you appreciate about your body each day	Did you meet the "no sugar" challenge? If not – what was your roadblock? check one roadblock?
1. _____	1 Yes__ No__ _____
2. _____	2 Yes__ No__ _____
3. _____	3 Yes__ No__ _____
4. _____	4 Yes__ No__ _____
5. _____	5 Yes__ No__ _____
6. _____	6 Yes__ No__ _____
7. _____	7 Yes__ No__ _____
8. _____	8 Yes__ No__ _____
9. _____	9 Yes__ No__ _____
10. _____	10. Yes__ No__ _____
11 _____	11 Yes__ No__ _____
12. _____	12. Yes__ No__ _____
13. _____	13. Yes__ No__ _____
14. _____	14. Yes__ No__ _____

Notes _____
_____
_____

Ready, Set, Goal!

Show that body some LOVE by crowding out sugar!

Page 11   (For Daughter)

Write down one thing you will appreciate about your body each day for the next two weeks.	Did you meet the "no sugar" challenge? If not – what was your roadblock? check one roadblock?
1. _____	1. Yes__ No__ _____
2. _____	2. Yes__ No__ _____
3. _____	3. Yes__ No__ _____
4. _____	4. Yes__ No__ _____
5. _____	5. Yes__ No__ _____
6. _____	6. Yes__ No__ _____
7. _____	7. Yes__ No__ _____
8. _____	8. Yes__ No__ _____
9. _____	9. Yes__ No__ _____
10. _____	10. Yes__ No__ _____
11. _____	11. Yes__ No__ _____
12. _____	12. Yes__ No__ _____
13. _____	13. Yes__ No__ _____
14. _____	14. Yes__ No__ _____

Notes _____

_____

_____

Support & Report

To be done on Day 14:
It's time for show & tell!
Review your Goal Sheets together

Page 12

Accountability CTA (Call to Action)

This is a time for celebration and reflection. You learned a lot in the past two weeks. You talked about some difficult subjects together and discovered some treasures in yourself and each other. It was the ideal first step in preparing you for the weeks to come. You are now armed with the awareness of your valuable body and your desire to treat it with gratitude and kindness. You are nurturing your body as you crowd out sugar with nutrient-dense foods. As you continue to model positive body talk and keep each other accountable, review what you've both learned and what you would like to improve upon. Consider your successes and your roadblocks.

Make a journal entry below to record these thoughts. Work together as you compile this entry. Well done, girls! It is time for your next module!

Notes _____

Whole Foods & Swap Outs

Learning to read labels & combat insulin resistance

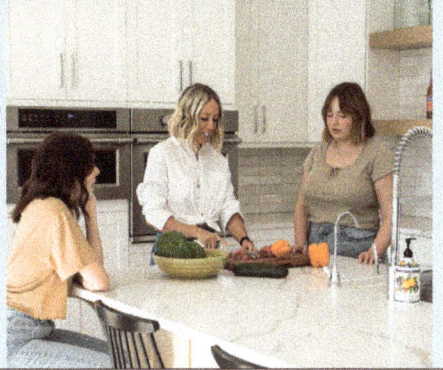

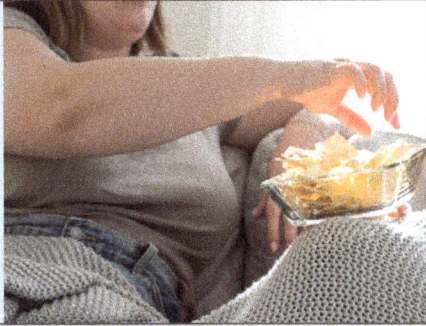

Welcome to Module #2! Your mother-daughter team is well on its way to metabolic wellness! It is time we learn about the pitfalls of highly processed, industrialized foods and the benefits of swapping them out for whole, organic options. This will help to reduce inflammation, which plays a crucial role in many health issues.

Topics in this Module

- Combat cravings
- Understand leveraging nutrients
- Prioritizing protein & healthy fats
- Shared experiences & growth

Transitioning to whole foods positively impacts our hormonal balance, aiding in weight management and easing symptoms of depression and anxiety. Prioritizing protein and whole foods helps combat various health concerns while providing sustainable energy and controlling cravings. When our nutritional needs are met, our body stops the search for nutrients, resulting in diminished cravings and satiety (feeling satisfied). Cheers to embracing this nutritious path together!

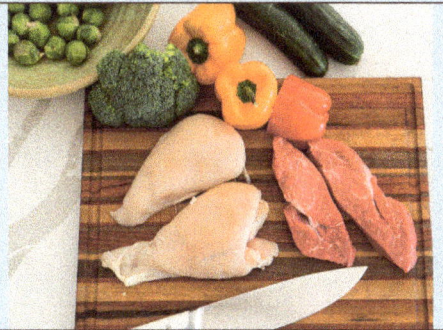

Notes _____

_____

_____

Time to Learn

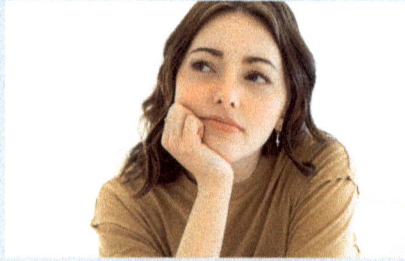

Page 1

What's Insulin Resistance?

Insulin resistance is when the cells in your body do not respond well to insulin, a hormone that regulates blood sugar. A few culprits go hand-in-hand with insulin resistance. For example, carrying extra weight, especially around the belly, or avoiding daily movement. Diets high in processed foods, sugar, and inflammatory ingredients can contribute to insulin resistance and can lead to obesity, type 2 Diabetes, Alzheimer's, heart disease, cancer, and hormone imbalances. This is not just happening to moms, daughters are not immune! PCOS (Polycystic Ovary Syndrome) is now considered a crisis on the rise of our younger generation. Obesity and type 2 diabetes are now common in children under age 10. Insulin resistance is directly linked to these diseases.

The Good News

As mom and daughter, you are on the path to healing. Together, you can take the steps to understand and support each other in your different life stages as you learn how insulin resistance can be prevented and managed! Encourage each other toward a healthy lifestyle with exercise desired for different stages - even just taking a walk, dancing to your favorite tunes, bike riding, hiking, or resistance training can make a big difference. Eating a protein-rich diet with loads of veggies, organic foods, and fiber and cutting back on added sugars and processed foods helps a bunch. Keeping an eye on your fat stores and prioritizing muscle growth will enhance your body's use of fuel and restore metabolic flexibility as you promote insulin sensitivity. Stress and sleep deprivation can also play a role in keeping insulin resistance rampant. A few simple changes can make a big difference in keeping your body high-functioning, beautiful vessels.

Notes _____

_____

_____

Time to Learn

Cravings and The Dorito Effect

Have you ever wondered why our bodies often go gaga for sugar and those ultra-processed, deliciously addictive snacks? It's called the "Dorito Effect" – these foods are engineered to make us crave more. A team of scientists, doctors, and consumers are brought in, and extensive studies are done that play with dopamine and satiety. By manufacturing a product with absolutely NO nutritional value but creating an intense dopamine hit, they've hit their jackpot! You are going to consume the entire bag, just like the commercial promises, because your body is not going to reach any state of satiety. After all, it's not receiving any nutrients. This causes intense cravings and hunger! But fear not! We have ways to tackle these cravings without feeling like we are missing out!

1. **Brain and Sugar Cravings:** Our brains adore the quick energy sugar and highly processed carbs provide, especially when we are not meeting our nutritional needs. The body will continue the search! The fix? Opt for protein and other whole foods, healthy fats, and fiber-rich meals. Snacks should never be just carbohydrates. Try to skip the snacks and satisfy your body's nutritional needs with the suggested choices to avoid the need for quick energy like carbs and sugar. You will be surprised how this tactic diminishes your cravings.

2. **Emotional Triggers:** Stress, boredom, or habit can push us toward these goodies. The commercialized food industry constantly tells us we need them! The solution? Check yourself when you go for a snack. What emotion are you feeling,? Do you normally snack at a certain time? Chances are, your body already has the fuel it needs, and this is an emotional desire. Find other ways to handle stress or emotions. You can pinpoint the emotion and write it down, take a walk, take deep breaths, or Facetime a friend. Grab a glass of water and talk it out. A good chat can beat a bag of chips any day!

3. **Microbiome and Cravings:** Our gut buddies have a say too! A diet heavy in these foods can influence gut bacteria, making us crave more of the same. The trick? Try eating 30 different types of food a week. High protein and fermented foods such as low-sugar yogurt, sauerkraut & kimchi support populating the gut microbiome, helping to balance those cravings. It's time to explore some new foods. You will never know if this really works until you test it out yourselves!

Notes _____

_____

_____

Time to Learn

The Magic of Prioritizing Protein

Let's dive into the fantastic world of protein and why it is like the superhero of our meals. Ever heard of the protein leverage hypothesis theory? It is the study that suggests our bodies, craving a specific amount of protein, end up overeating in search of it. Prioritizing protein in every meal might just be the secret sauce to boosting muscle mass, shedding unwanted fat, and keeping our metabolism in tip-top shape. It is like our meal's VIP guest, making everything better!

1. **Power-Up with Protein**: Swapping processed munchies for whole foods loaded with protein helps in various ways. For instance, instead of those sugary cereal bars, try Greek yogurt or a handful of nuts. Protein's muscle-building superpower keeps you feeling fuller for longer, reducing the urge to snack constantly. Plus, it is like a secret fat-burning code—more protein means the body burns more energy digesting it! It is called the thermic effect of food (TEF). When eating foods that rank higher in thermogenesis, your body will burn about 20% more fuel as it digests. This is great news for your metabolism.

2. **Smart Protein Swaps**: Ditching processed foods like low-grade sausages or deli meats, opt for grass-fed or free range when possible. It is not just about saying 'no' to processed items; it is about saying 'yes' to a whole squad of nutrients. Real foods keep us satisfied and pack a punch with healthy nutrients, unlike the empty promises, added hormones, and toxins from processed or industrialized protein sources.

3. **Balance it Right**: Instead of relying on industrialized processed shakes or bars, blend up a protein-packed smoothie with whole ingredients like spinach, berries, and a scoop of high-quality, grass-fed protein powder (preferably whey protein isolate vs concentrate). Not only does this keep those muscles happy by stimulating muscle protein synthesis, but it also gives your body a full spectrum of amino acids it needs to build and repair cells daily. Again - another metabolism booster!

Notes _____
_____
_____

Page 4 Time to Learn

The First Thing to Swap is Your Oils

The following oils, PUFAs, are polyunsaturated fatty acids. When PUFAs oxidize, they can generate free radicals, leading to inflammation and potentially contributing to various health problems. When the body endures this oxidative stress, it cannot release unwanted fat.

Oils OUT

Canola oil	Cotton Seed	Corn oil	Safflower oil
Sunflower oil	Rapeseed oil	Vegetable oil	Soybean oil

Replace WITH

Olive oil	Avocado oil	Coconut oil
Real Butter	Tallow or Lard	Peanut oil

7 Highly Processed Foods to Swap Out

Artificial ingredients

1: This includes both synthetic dyes (like FD&C Red No. 40, Tartrazine, or Blue No. 1) and artificial sweeteners (like saccharin, aspartame, or sucralose). Artificial dyes require a warning label in many countries outside of the U.S. This is enough of an indicator for us at EmpowHer!

Instead: Look for dyes that come from natural sources (like paprika, saffron, or annatto) or forget the coloring all together (it's only for aesthetics). When it comes to sweeteners pick those that come from natural sources (like honey, maple syrup, and even sugar) over the artificial stuff, but always consume them in moderation. They still raise your blood sugar and insulin levels.

Notes _____

_____

_____

Time to Learn

Refined Sweeteners

2. It's not that refined sweeteners themselves (like sugar) are completely bad, but the quantity in which sweeteners are consumed these days is honestly the scary part. Sugar (or corn syrup or cane juice or brown rice syrup or whatever creative name is on the label) is no longer reserved for truly special occasions anymore, and instead is lurking in yogurts, breads, crackers, flavored oatmeal, beverages, and even innocent-looking salad dressings.

Instead: Rely on natural sweeteners like honey and maple syrup since they are mostly "processed" in nature and at least contain some trace nutrients. BUT it is important to remember that "sugar is sugar" no matter what you choose. So even if you go the more natural route (which is recommended!) that by no means gives you the green light.

Refined Grains

3. This includes products made from white flour (usually labeled as enriched "wheat" flour), white rice, corn meal, etc. When grains are refined, the most nutritional part of the grain (the bran and germ) is removed. This prolongs shelf life, among other things, but remember...real food should (and does!) rot, so avoid the science experiment and stick to the whole grains provided to us by nature.

Instead: Give up the white stuff and rely on nutritious whole grains like whole-wheat flour, oats, brown rice, quinoa, and others. Or go gluten-free with almond or coconut flour.

Factory-Farmed Meat and Seafood

4. Animals raised in incredibly crowded and confined quarters likely never see the light of day. What's more, these animals are often fed unnatural diets. Including synthetic hormones and antibiotics to ensure they produce the most abundant meat products as quickly and efficiently as possible. Animals raised in such an unhealthy environment produce products that are not as nutritious for you as the local, pastured (or wild-caught) alternatives. Better nutrition = better satiety.

Instead: Try shopping at your local farmers' market for grass-fed, pastured animal products. If you enjoy fish, search out the "wild-caught" variety.

Notes

Time to Learn

Ingredients You Would Not Cook with at Home

5. Rather than memorizing a complicated list of chemicals to avoid in packaged foods, I will make this really easy for you. Do not buy anything packaged that is made with ingredients you would not cook with at home. These are fillers, emulsifiers, and preservatives (which are usually items you can not even pronounce). They lack nutrients, cause inflammation, and immense cravings. Your body will continue to search for the lacking nutrients (Remember the Doritos!).

Instead: Stick with simple products made from a handful of pure ingredients. The fewer ingredients the better! Or make food yourself from scratch at home, a perfect activity for mom and daughter.

Imitation Foods

6. This includes anything trying to pretend to be something it is not. Margarine (or vegan "butter"), processed cheese products, imitation crab meat, pancake "syrup," and "lemonade" powder are all great examples. It is up to you to not only read the front of the packaging but flip it over and search for the ingredients on the back. Look at all you are learning and all the inflammation you are avoiding!

Instead: Buy the "real" versions of foods like real butter, real cheese, real crab, or pure maple syrup, and make lemonade with real lemons (not artificial powder!).

Low-Fat and Fat-Free Products

7. You are off the hook. "Diet" foods are not only more processed to get the fat out, but they never tasted that good anyway! As it turns out, we have gotten fat on low-fat products. And that is because when they take the fat out of these foods they no longer taste good so they have to add in a bunch of sugar. Binging on sugar and other refined sweeteners is the real issue here...not eating healthy fats.

Instead: Switch to full-fat dairy, including milk, and avoid low-fat packaged foods altogether. Healthy fats are great for our brain and hormonal function, they also do not spike your blood sugar and insulin!

Notes _____

_____

_____

Pen to Paper

It's time to go to work!

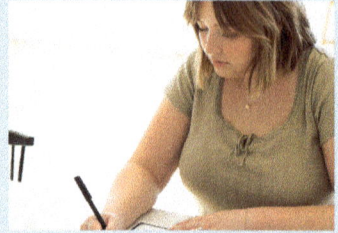

Daughter's Worksheet

Are you showing signs of Insulin Resistance?

Do you have stubborn weight around your midsection? No matter how much you exercise or cut calories, this weight is determined to stay!

○ ___Not at all___   ○ ___Somewhat___   ○ ___More than average___

Do you have cravings for immediate fuel, such as sugar or processed carbohydrates, even when you know you shouldn't be hungry? When blood sugar starts to decline, our body wants immediate fuel to increase our energy levels. You might be stuck in sugar-burning mode vs the ability to use fat as fuel.

○ ___Not at all___   ○ ___Somewhat___   ○ ___More than average___

Do you have noticeable energy dips? Our bodies were never meant for grazing. Going without food for a period of time shouldn't leave you feeling tired. Many complain of brain fog or lack of concentration.

○ ___Not at all___   ○ ___Somewhat___   ○ ___More than average___

Do you have trouble sleeping? There are many factors that cause sleep trouble. Insulin resistance causes hormone imbalances that contribute to sleep disruption.

○ ___Not at all___   ○ ___Somewhat___   ○ ___More than average___

Do you struggle with gut issues? Often times our resistance to insulin has increased due to choosing packaged, highly processed foods. These foods are known to cause inflammation and leaky gut. Bloating, pain, and digestive issues are common in those with insulin resistance.

○ ___Not at all___   ○ ___Somewhat___   ○ ___More than average___

Notes _____

_____

_____

Pen to Paper

It's time to go to work!

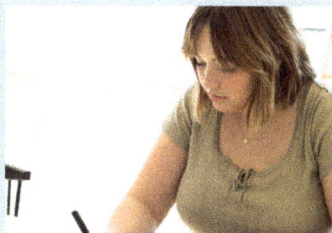

Mom's Worksheet

Are you showing
signs of Insulin
Resistance?

Do you have stubborn weight around your midsection? No matter how much you exercise or cut calories, this weight is determined to stay!

○ _____ Not at all   ○ _____ Somewhat   ○ _____ More than average

Do you have cravings for immediate fuel, such as sugar or processed carbohydrates, even when you know you shouldn't be hungry? When blood sugar starts to decline, our body wants immediate fuel to increase our energy levels. You might be stuck in sugar-burning mode vs the ability to use fat as fuel.

○ _____ Not at all   ○ _____ Somewhat   ○ _____ More than average

Do you have noticeable energy dips? Our bodies were never meant for grazing. Going without food for a period of time shouldn't leave you feeling tired. Many complain of brain fog or lack of concentration.

○ _____ Not at all   ○ _____ Somewhat   ○ _____ More than average

Do you have trouble sleeping? There are many factors that cause sleep trouble. Insulin resistance causes hormone imbalances that contribute to sleep disruption.

○ _____ Not at all   ○ _____ Somewhat   ○ _____ More than average

Do you struggle with gut issues? Often times our resistance to insulin has increased due to choosing packaged, highly processed foods. These foods are known to cause inflammation and leaky gut. Bloating, pain, and digestive issues are common in those with insulin resistance.

○ _____ Not at all   ○ _____ Somewhat   ○ _____ More than average

Notes _____

_____

_____

Ready, Set, Goal!

It's time for some self-reflection & goal-setting!

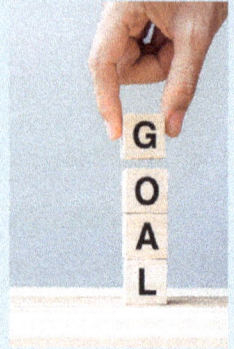

Page 9

Summary

If you scored 3 or more answers with "somewhat" or above, you are probably beginning to show signs of insulin resistance. Do not panic. Over 88% of Americans show some signs of metabolic disease. Congratulations on being one of the 3% of Americans who actually do something about it! Well done.

Insulin resistance is more than struggling to lose weight. It can lead to serious conditions like obesity, diabetes, heart disease, liver disease, and Alzheimer's.

Although the previous checklist is something to consider when determining insulin resistance, there are metabolic blood panels that can be done to find more definitive answers to your concerns. These tests will include helpful information such as fasting insulin levels, fasting glucose, and Hemoglobin A1C.

Insulin resistance results when your body can't process insulin properly. Diet, lack of exercise, stress, and toxins increase your levels of insulin resistance. Functional medicine seeks to address these aggravators so your body is better able to process insulin and use it better.

With a functional coaching plan, you address some of the potential causes of the disease. Instead of treating symptoms, you revise the habits that cause the dysfunction in the first place.

If you're diagnosed with Type 2 diabetes, prediabetes, or PCOS, you have options for treatment that do not involve medications and insulin pumps. Committing to the practices in this module as you revise your diet and specific exercises can support a reversal of insulin resistance. A diagnosis from your doctor and support from a Functional Health Coach are the perfect path for mom and daughter empowerment!

Notes _____

_____

_____

Ready, Set, Goal!

Prioritizing Protein

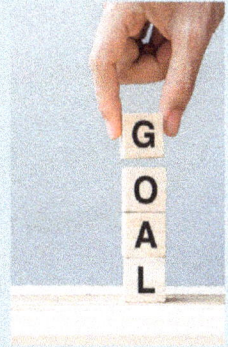

Page 10

You'll both have a goal sheet that will require daily reflection and a record of your experience surrounding prioritizing protein and swapping out for nutrient-dense foods. Keep the following information in mind when meeting these goals.

You will be asked to "prioritize protein." Here is why:

Eating 30 grams of protein per meal is like fueling your body with superpowers! Studies show it significantly amps up metabolism, keeping your body's energy-burning furnace revved. With this threshold dose, you will notice fewer cravings as it keeps you feeling full longer as your nutritional needs are being met. Protein is a muscle-building beast, supporting strong and healthy lean muscle tissue. Protein helps keep you steady all day by diminishing hunger hormones like ghrelin and lowering insulin levels. So, 30 grams of protein is not just a number on your plate. It is a powerful secret to optimizing your health, shedding some fat while supporting your metabolic rate, and feeling awesome! Believe it or not, you will not even have to count calories. Just make sure you're hitting your 30 grams per meal, and you will be amazed at what happens. Trust me ladies!

HELPFUL Hints

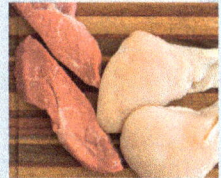

- Chicken 4.7 oz = 30 g
- Ground beef 6 oz = 30 g
- Turkey breast 4.5 oz = 30 g
- Pork tenderloin 5.3 oz = 30 g
- Wild Salmon 5.3 oz = 30 g
- Cod 6 oz = 30 g
- Shrimp 5.3 oz = 30 g
- Top sirloin steak 4.8 oz = 30 g
- Lambchop 5.7 oz = 30 g
- Oikos Pro Greek yogurt 3/4 c = 25 g
- Cottage cheese 1 c = 26 g
- 1 Egg = 6 g
- Average protein powder 1 scoop = 25 g

Notes _____

_____

_____

Ready, Set, Goal!

Let's Swap!

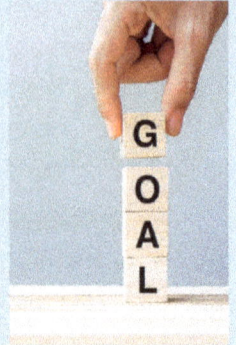

Page 11

As you support each other to make healthy, whole-food swaps, it is important to remember that you can not fix everything at once! Each day, you will be encouraged to swap out something less nutrient-dense with a "cleaner" version. Put aside the foods you have learned cause inflammation, weight-loss resistance, hormonal imbalances, and immense cravings.

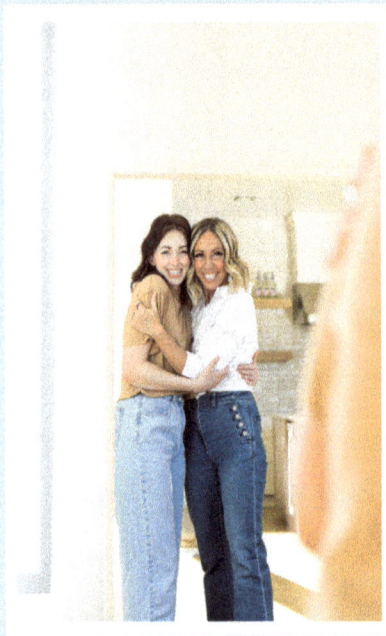

You will be asked to swap out the "yuck" for the "luck." Here is why:

If you want to swap out your whole pantry in one day – go for it! As for this week's goal – we will only require you to record one item a day. You can go to the store and find similar replacements – or find completely new, whole-food choices. You will discover that your cravings for highly palatable processed foods diminish as you feed your body the nutrients it craves. This will be a fun project to tackle together. If you do not live close to each other, send pictures of the item you find. It is like a treasure hunt to find clean, wholesome foods in a grocery store! Remember to refer to the material in this module as you seek out these swaps. Learning this skill sets you far ahead of the game when it comes to true lifestyle change and sustainable metabolic health!

Notes _____

_____

_____

Ready, Set, Goal!

Swap out and
prioritize protein

Page 12   **For Mom**

Write down one thing you swapped out and what you replaced it with each day.		Did you meet the "30 g of protein/meal" challenge? If not – what was your roadblock?	
old choice	new choice	check one	roadblock?
1. _____	for	1. Yes__ No__	_____
2. _____	for	2. Yes__ No__	_____
3. _____	for	3. Yes__ No__	_____
4. _____	for	4. Yes__ No__	_____
5. _____	for	5. Yes__ No__	_____
6. _____	for	6. Yes__ No__	_____
7. _____	for	7. Yes__ No__	_____
8. _____	for	8. Yes__ No__	_____
9. _____	for	9. Yes__ No__	_____
10. _____	for	10. Yes__ No__	_____
11. _____	for	11. Yes__ No__	_____
12. _____	for	12. Yes__ No__	_____
13. _____	for	13. Yes__ No__	_____
14. _____	for	14. Yes__ No__	_____

Notes _____

_____

_____

Ready, Set, Goal!

Swap out and prioritize protein

Page 13

For Daughter

Write down one thing you swapped out and what you replaced it with each day.		Did you meet the "30 g of protein/meal" challenge? If not – what was your roadblock?	
old choice	new choice	check one	roadblock?
1. _____	for	1. Yes__ No__ _____	
2. _____	for	2. Yes__ No__ _____	
3. _____	for	3. Yes__ No__ _____	
4. _____	for	4. Yes__ No__ _____	
5. _____	for	5. Yes__ No__ _____	
6. _____	for	6. Yes__ No__ _____	
7. _____	for	7. Yes__ No__ _____	
8. _____	for	8. Yes__ No__ _____	
9. _____	for	9. Yes__ No__ _____	
10. _____	for	10. Yes__ No__ _____	
11. _____	for	11. Yes__ No__ _____	
12. _____	for	12. Yes__ No__ _____	
13. _____	for	13. Yes__ No__ _____	
14. _____	for	14. Yes__ No__ _____	

Notes _____
_____
_____

Support & Report

To be done on Day 14:

It's time for show & tell!

Review your Goal Sheets together

Page 14

Accountability CTA (call To Action)

This is a time for celebration and reflection. You have made some important lifestyle changes these past two weeks. Changes this significant can be hard! As you have learned the possibilities of finding freedom from sugar and highly processed food addictions, you have seen how your body can react when given the nutrients it needs. If your goals include shedding fat and preventing disease, these strategies will get the job done. These are lifelong tools you will both use in supporting each other and sharing with your family as you continue on your journey.

It is now time to stop and reflect. How did it go? What did you find most challenging? Was there anything that surprised you? What is the most valuable thing you learned in Module #2? What is something you wish you had done differently? What are you most proud of? Take this time to collaborate. Write down your thoughts as you answer these prompts together. Get ready – It is almost for your next module!

Notes

Rest & Digest Metabolic Reset

The benefits of time-restricted eating to support metabolic flexibility

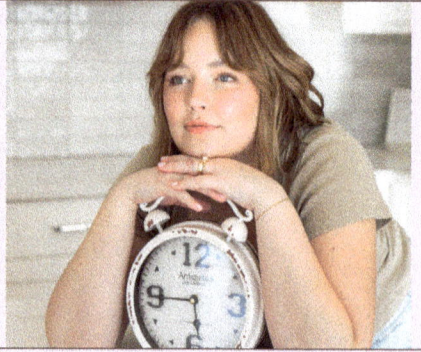

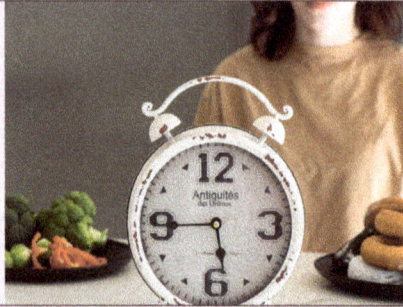

Welcome to Module #3. Your mother-daughter team is ready to learn the science of time-restricted eating. We will delve into the science and its impact on metabolic health. We will explore the benefits of eating during a specific time window, enhancing insulin sensitivity, reducing sugar cravings, and promoting metabolic freedom to enhance overall health.

Topics in this Module

- Teach your body to use fat as fuel
- The benefits of lowering insulin levels
- Disease prevention & metabolic health
- Shared experiences & growth

Shifting from sugar burning to fat burning is crucial for sustained energy, improved body composition, and disease prevention. Insulin resistance, a key factor in obesity and diseases, is addressed through time-restricted eating. By embracing this method, your bodies will become more insulin-sensitive, promoting efficient energy utilization and reducing the risk of health issues. Together, let's cultivate habits that foster well-being and metabolic resilience for a sustainable lifestyle.

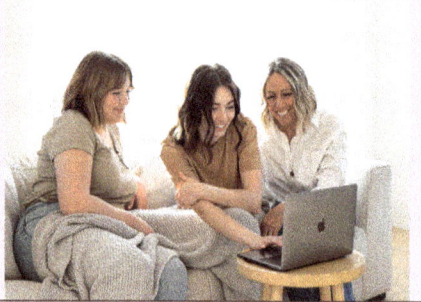

Notes _____

_____

_____

Time to Learn

Page 1

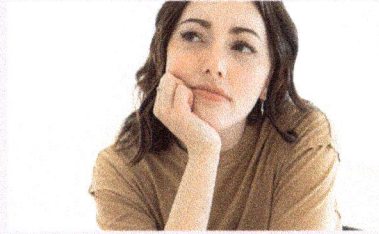

Using Time-Restricted Eating to Become Fat-Adapted:

Hello, moms and daughters! It is time to talk about becoming fat-adapted and unlocking a world of energy and health. Time-restricted eating can be a secret weapon, teaching our bodies to be efficient fat burners. This approach is a game-changer, especially in a world that encourages most of our food to come from sources that raise our insulin levels and lock up our most crucial fuel, fat! By moving our eating to specific time windows, we shift our metabolism. During fasting periods, our bodies tap into fat stores for energy, making us efficient fat burners. This process enhances insulin sensitivity, a key player in weight management and overall health. When we are fat-adapted, our bodies become skilled at using fat as a primary fuel source, promoting weight loss and improving metabolic health.

The Magic:

Imagine the empowerment that comes with knowing our bodies are adaptable powerhouses! It is like turning on a switch that says, "Hey, body, let's use fat for fuel!" Time-restricted eating is not a diet or about deprivation, it is quite the opposite. It encourages a lifestyle that offers higher energy levels and less cravings. It lowers our blood sugar and insulin as we use ketones (fat) as fuel! Time-restricted eating is not about saying "no" to delicious meals. It is about saying "yes" at the right times. **It is not about eating less. It is about eating less often.** This approach nurtures a beautiful relationship with food, allowing our bodies to focus on digestion during specific windows. It is a journey towards mindful eating, creating a space for us to savor each bite and celebrate the nourishment it brings.

Notes _____

_____

_____

Time to Learn

How to Get Started

To start time-restricted eating, align with the sun's natural cycle (circadian rhythm) for a 12-hour fast. When the sun goes down or after dinner, shut off your digestion and stop eating. During this time avoid anything causing an insulin response, even minor flavors or bites (like lemon in water), to grant your body complete rest from digestion. To sustain a fasted state, continue drinking water and even add some sea salt for electrolyte balance and optimal hydration. **For those over 18,** focus on promoting autophagy, which is the cleaning up of damaged cells and promoting cell renewal. Autophagy can occur at about 15-17 hours. Next, you will focus on insulin sensitivity— slowly working up to longer fasts if you feel. Embrace fat adaptation through longer fasts, enhancing the body's ability to burn fat efficiently as insulin levels decrease. Stay hydrated to support metabolic processes and manage hunger. Incorporate exercise to boost fat utilization and preserve muscle mass during fasting. **Growing adolescents should be cautious and not exceed 11-12 hours.** A little intentional stress on the body is good! Be mindful that too much fasting too soon can cause a fight or flight stress response and feelings of deprivation. This should be avoided. Remember, as mom and daughter, we are on this journey to nurture, love, and care for our bodies. This mindset is most important for our overall health.

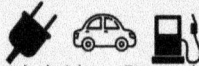

Fat for Fuel Analogy: Imagine driving a hybrid car. It runs by using 50 miles of electrical energy and 500 miles from burning gasoline. Let's say we plug it in after every 50 miles. This would mean we never get into the gasoline stored in the gas tank. This is what happens to our body when we eat every few hours during the day. We never get into our fat stores because we continue to use sugar/glucose. Our insulin levels stay elevated and we lock up our fat stores. Time-restricted eating teaches our body to make the metabolic switch and use fat as an energy source.

Enhanced Hormonal Sensitivity: Time-restricted eating helps to improve insulin sensitivity. Insulin acts as a master regulator of hormone signaling. Lowering insulin levels enhances the sensitivity of cells to other hormones, including those that regulate reproductive health and metabolism. This improved sensitivity can positively impact menstrual regularity and fertility in women. Insulin influences the production of sex hormones, such as estrogen and testosterone. Lowering insulin levels helps maintain a more balanced ratio of these hormones, which is crucial for reproductive health, mood regulation, and overall hormonal equilibrium. Both mothers and daughters, while in different hormonal stages in life, benefit from hormonal balance. Lowering insulin through lifestyle interventions like fasting, regular exercise, and mindful eating can promote hormonal harmony. This will positively impact weight, blood sugar levels, inflammation, and reproductive health. We are on our way to metabolic freedom by using tools like time-restricted eating in our lifestyle toolkit. Supporting each other as we practice this new skill will bring great empowerment!

Notes _____

_____

_____

Time to Learn

Breaking a fast is a crucial step that should be done mindfully to avoid digestive discomfort and to optimize the benefits of fasting. Here are some general guidelines on how to break a fast and what to eat during your eating window:

Breaking the Fast:

1. Start with Simple: Hydrate your body with water first. A good bone broth tea is healing for the gut lining. Once you see your gut does not react, continue to eat your healthy choices.
2. Incorporate Probiotics: Consider including probiotic-rich foods or supplements to promote gut health. Options include yogurt, kefir, sauerkraut, or a high-quality probiotic supplement.
3. Choose Easily Digestible Foods: Begin with easily digestible foods like a small serving of cooked vegetables or broth. This helps to reintroduce nutrients to your digestive system gently.
4. Include Proteins: Continue to prioritize protein sources such as grilled chicken, fish, tofu, beef, and pork. Protein helps rebuild tissues and supports and maintains muscle health.
5. Healthy Fats: Incorporate healthy fats, like avocados, coconut oil, or olive oil, to provide sustained energy and support various bodily functions.

During the Eating Window:

1. Macronutrients: Strive to prioritize your protein. Let a healthy mix of natural carbohydrates and healthy fats fill in the gaps.
2. Avoid Processed Foods: Minimize processed and refined foods. They can spike blood sugar levels and counteract some of the benefits of fasting.
3. Mindful Eating: Practice mindful eating by paying attention to hunger and fullness cues. Chew your food thoroughly and savor the flavors to enhance digestion.
4. Stay Hydrated: Continue to drink water throughout your eating window to stay hydrated. Herbal teas and infused electrolyte water are also good options.
5. Meal Timing: Depending on your fasting method, consider spacing out your meals during the eating window to maintain steady energy levels. Snacking unnecessarily raises blood sugar and insulin. Eating nutrient-dense meals should help you avoid the need for snacks.

Remember, individual dietary needs vary. What works for one person may not work for another. It is advisable to listen to your body and adjust your eating habits based on your specific health goals and preferences. If you have any existing health conditions or concerns, it is recommended to consult with a healthcare professional or a registered dietitian before making significant changes to your diet or fasting routine.

Notes

Time to Learn

What is Happening in My Body When I Fast?

Fasting triggers a series of physiological changes within your body, adapting it to the absence of food intake. Here is what typically happens during a fast:

Glycogen Depletion
Your body stores glucose as glycogen in the liver and muscles. In the initial hours of fasting, these glycogen stores are depleted. This is a quick source of energy, and its reduction signals the body to shift to alternative fuel sources.

Insulin Levels Drop
Fasting leads to a decrease in insulin levels. Insulin is a hormone that helps cells absorb glucose from the bloodstream. With lower insulin levels, your body becomes more efficient at burning fat for energy.

Ketosis Begins
As glycogen stores are depleted, the body starts breaking down fat into ketones, a process known as ketosis. These ketones become an alternative energy source, particularly for the brain and muscles.

Autophagy Activation
Fasting stimulates autophagy, a cellular recycling process where damaged or malfunctioning cellular components are broken down and removed. This helps in cellular repair and rejuvenation.

Hormone Regulation
Fasting influences the release of various hormones. Growth hormone increases, promoting muscle preservation and fat utilization. Noradrenaline and cortisol levels rise, enhancing alertness and the mobilization of energy reserves.

Cellular Repair & Regeneration
The body focuses on repairing and regenerating cells during fasting. This includes repairing damaged DNA, reducing oxidative stress, and promoting overall cellular health.

Blood Sugar Stabilization
Fasting can contribute to stabilizing blood sugar levels. The body becomes more efficient at using available glucose and relies on gluconeogenesis to produce glucose from non-carbohydrate sources like protein.

Notes _____

_____

_____

Time to Learn

Reduction in Inflammation
Fasting has been associated with a decrease in markers of inflammation. This anti-inflammatory effect contributes to the prevention of chronic diseases.

Improved Insulin Sensitivity
Over time, regular fasting improves insulin sensitivity, helping to regulate blood sugar levels and reduce the risk of insulin resistance, type 2 diabetes, Alzheimer's, heart disease, and obesity.

Enhanced Brain Function
Fasting has been linked to cognitive benefits, including improved brain function, increased BDNF (brain-derived neurotrophic factor), and potential protection against neurodegenerative diseases.

Other Types of Fasting

This list is for educational purposes. Although some of the following fasting methods are similar to time-restricted eating, we will not be using these fasting methods specifically in our EmpowerHer program. However, you may consult with your healthcare provider if you would like to try any of the following.

▷ Intermittent Fasting:
- Type: This involves cycling between periods of eating and fasting.
- Benefits: Improves insulin sensitivity, promotes weight loss, supports metabolic health, and may enhance longevity. Common methods include the 16/8 method (16 hours fasting, 8 hours eating) and the 5:2 method (eating normally for five days, restricting calorie intake on two non-consecutive days).

▷ Alternate-Day Fasting (ADF):
- Type: Alternating between days of normal eating and days of either very low-calorie intake or complete fasting.
- Benefits: Similar to intermittent fasting, it may lead to weight loss, improved insulin sensitivity, and reduced risk of chronic diseases. It can be challenging and may not be suitable for everyone.

Notes _____

_____

_____

Time to Learn

▷ Fasting–Mimicking Diet (FMD):
- Type: Consuming a diet that mimics the effects of fasting by providing low–calorie, plant–based foods for a limited duration.
- Benefits: Supports cellular regeneration, may reduce markers of aging, improves metabolic health, and has shown potential benefits in cancer prevention and treatment. The FMD allows for some food intake, making it more feasible for some individuals compared to complete fasting.

▷ Extended Fasting:
- Type: Fasting for an extended period, typically beyond 48 hours.
- Benefits: Promotes deeper autophagy, may enhance stem cell regeneration, and has been associated with increased mental clarity. Extended fasting requires careful planning and supervision due to potential risks, and it's not recommended for everyone.

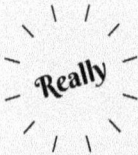

Really

Fasting is a Historical Practice: Interesting Fact

Pythagoras, the ancient Greek philosopher and mathematician, believed that abstaining from food could purify the body and mind, fostering clarity of thought and spiritual insight. His philosophy extended beyond mathematical principles to encompass a holistic approach to health. Pythagoras and his followers, known as the Pythagoreans, practiced dietary restrictions, including periods of fasting, as part of their commitment to a harmonious and disciplined lifestyle.

This historical perspective highlights the longstanding connection between fasting and philosophical or spiritual practices, emphasizing the belief that fasting not only has physical benefits but can also contribute to mental clarity and spiritual development. This is also why many major religions follow some type of fasting practice.

There must be something to it if it is still practiced among health and wellness advocates worldwide. As mom and daughter, let's embark on our fasting journey!

Notes _____

_____

_____

Pen to Paper

It's time to go to work!

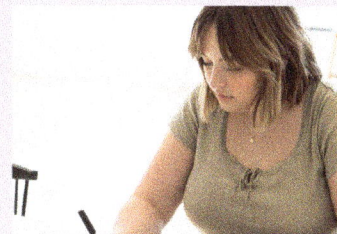

Daughter's Worksheet

1. **Motivation:**

Why are you interested in implementing time-restricted eating and narrowing your eating window?

What specific health or wellness goals do you hope to achieve through time-restricted eating?

2. **Current Lifestyle:**

How would you describe your current daily eating habits and patterns?

What challenges, if any, do you foresee in adjusting your eating window based on your current lifestyle?

3. **Awareness:**

How familiar are you with the concept of time-restricted eating?

How well do you understand the information about the potential benefits and challenges of time-restricted eating?

4. **Readiness:**

On a scale of 1 to 10, how ready do you feel to commit to a specific time-restricted eating schedule?

What factors might impact your ability to adhere to a time-restricted eating pattern?

5. **Support System:**

Do you have a support system (family, friends, etc.) that is aware of and supportive of your decision to time-restrict your eating window?

How do you plan to manage social situations or events that may involve eating outside your designated window?

Notes _____

_____

_____

Pen to Paper

It's time to go to work!

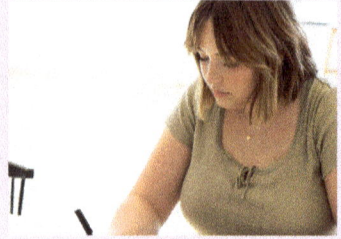

Mom's Worksheet

1. Motivation:
Why are you interested in implementing time-restricted eating and narrowing your eating window?

What specific health or wellness goals do you hope to achieve through time-restricted eating?

2. Current Lifestyle:
How would you describe your current daily eating habits and patterns?

What challenges, if any, do you foresee in adjusting your eating window based on your current lifestyle?

3. Awareness:
How familiar are you with the concept of time-restricted eating?

How well do you understand the information about the potential benefits and challenges of time-restricted eating?

4. Readiness:
On a scale of 1 to 10, how ready do you feel to commit to a specific time-restricted eating schedule?

What factors might impact your ability to adhere to a time-restricted eating pattern?

5. Support System:
Do you have a support system (family, friends, etc.) that is aware of and supportive of your decision to time-restrict your eating window?

How do you plan to manage social situations or events that may involve eating outside your designated window?

Notes _____

_____

_____

Ready, Set, Goal!

It's time for some self-reflection & goal-setting!

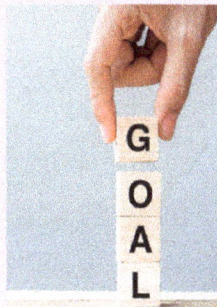

Page 9

Summary

Let's delve into the questions and explore the possible answers, deciphering what they might reveal about you and your daughter embarking on the journey of time-restricted eating.

1. Motivation:
- Possible Answers:
  - You might have expressed a desire for weight management, improved energy levels, or enhanced overall well-being.
  - Or you might have cited specific health concerns, such as insulin sensitivity or metabolic health.
- Interpretation:
  - Strong motivations suggest a clear understanding of personal health goals, indicating that you are likely committed and focused on achieving positive outcomes through time-restricted eating. This clarity can serve as a powerful driver for success.

2. Current Lifestyle:
- Possible Answers:
  - Your response may range from irregular eating patterns to consistent three-meals-a-day habits.
  - Or you might have highlighted challenges like irregular work hours or frequent social engagements involving food.
- Interpretation:
  - Understanding current habits and challenges provides insights into potential adjustments needed for successful time-restricted eating. It helps to recognize these challenges to tailor your approach to this lifestyle, making it more practical and sustainable.

3. Awareness:
- Possible Answers:
  - You may have indicated varying levels of familiarity with time-restricted eating, from detailed research to a general awareness.
  - Or you might have expressed curiosity but admit that you have limited knowledge.
- Interpretation:
  - A higher awareness level suggests you have sought information and likely understand the principles and potential benefits of time-restricted eating. For those less familiar, education is crucial. Please read closely over this Module until you understand the methods and benefits of time-restricted eating.

4. Readiness:
- Possible Answers:
  - You might have expressed high readiness, indicating enthusiasm and confidence in adopting time-restricted eating.
  - Or you might have scored lower, indicating hesitation, concerns, or need more information.
- Interpretation:
  - High readiness signals a strong willingness to make changes, while lower scores suggest potential barriers that need addressing. Understanding readiness, knowledge, and motivation helps tailor and ensure the transition is gradual and manageable.

5. Support System:
- Possible Answers:
  - You may have a supportive network aware of and encouraging your health journey.
  - Or you might have expressed concerns about potential resistance or lack of understanding from those around you.
- Interpretation:
  - A strong support system can significantly contribute to success in time-restricted eating. Awareness of potential challenges in social situations allows for proactive strategies to navigate those scenarios effectively.

The responses to these questions paint a picture of your readiness and potential challenges in adopting time-restricted eating. A strong motivation, coupled with an understanding of current habits and potential obstacles, sets the stage for a more tailored and sustainable approach. It also highlights the importance of education and support, ensuring that you are well-equipped to embark on this dietary journey. Ultimately, the goal is to foster a positive and realistic mindset, making time-restricted eating not just a temporary change but a sustainable and beneficial lifestyle choice.

Notes _____

_____

_____

Ready, Set, Goal!

Start the Rest & Digest Timer

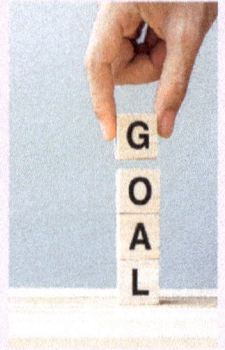

Page 10

You will both have a goal sheet that will require daily reflection and a record of your experience surrounding time-restricted eating with recorded cut-off times and eating windows. Keep the following information in mind when meeting these goals.

You will be asked to record your eating and fasting windows along with your total hours fasted. Here is why.

Embarking on time-restricted eating involves a gradual and mindful approach. Start by hydrating well before the fast to mitigate potential side effects. When beginning your time-restricted period, abstain from any food or beverages, relying solely on water for hydration. This exclusion is crucial to avoid triggering insulin release or elevated blood sugar levels, compromising the fasting benefits.

The essence of resting your digestive and other body systems lies in inducing a parasympathetic state, where the body prioritizes repair and regeneration. This state facilitates autophagy, the cellular cleaning process, and depletes glycogen stores, prompting a metabolic shift towards fat utilization for energy—a key component of metabolic flexibility.

During the fast, listen to your body and stay attuned to signs of hunger or fatigue. Remember to start slow and low. If under 18, attune your rest and digest times with your natural circadian rhythm, which aligns with the setting and rising of the sun. Consulting with a healthcare professional before embarking on any fast, especially for extended durations, is advisable.

Approaching a fast with mindfulness will maximize its potential benefits while prioritizing overall health and well-being.

HELPFUL Hints

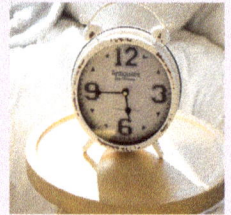

- Remember to eat enough
- It is not about eating less – just less often
- Continue to choose whole foods
- Continue to crowd out sugar
- Continue to crowd out processed carbs
- Prioritize protein (aim for 30 g/meal)
- Add in healthy fats
- Stay hydrated
- Keep your electrolytes balanced
- Add some sea salt to your water
- Sneaking in bites /tastes will cause hunger
- Take it slow when you begin eating
- Listen to your body's cues

Notes _____

_____

_____

Ready, Set, Goal!

Let's Eat!

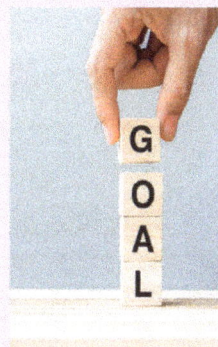

Page 11

As you support each other with time-restricted eating, it is important to remember that you will need time to adjust! Each day, you will feel a shift and notice different hunger responses and energy levels. Be encouraged as you note these changes. Your body is learning to become more efficient and intuitive. To optimize your fasting period, fill your eating window with the nutrient-dense foods we have been focusing on. Remember, it is not about calorie restriction – it is time restriction.

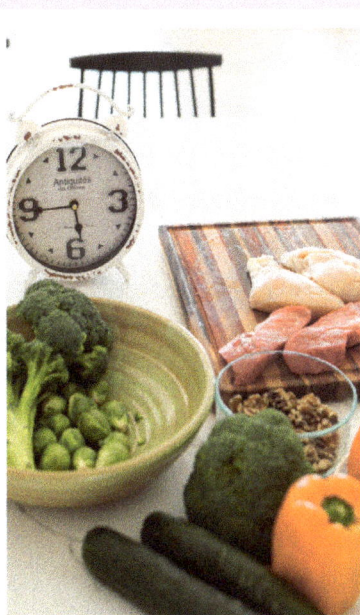

You will be asked to end your time-restricted eating or fast with ease as your body adjusts. You will also take note if you met the rest and digest challenge each day and record any road blocks you may have encountered.

Ending a fast requires gradual reintroduction of food to avoid digestive discomfort. The body becomes more intuitive post-fast, so be attentive to reactions. Start with easily digestible, nutrient-dense foods like protein, healthy fats and vegetables, aiding the digestive system's gentle transition. Optimize fasting benefits by filling the eating window with whole, nutrient-rich foods, promoting cellular repair and metabolic health. If unsure about a particular food or beverage affecting the fasting state, consume it during the eating window. Medications should be taken as prescribed, irrespective of fasting, to ensure health needs are met. This mindful approach to breaking a fast enhances the overall fasting experience and fosters sustained well-being. Always consult with a healthcare professional for personalized advice, especially if dealing with specific health conditions. Let's eat!

Notes _____

_____

_____

Ready, Set, Goal!

Rest and Digest
+ Refuel Time

Page 12 (For Mom)

Record the time you stop eating and when you begin to refuel. Take note of the total time fasted.				Did you meet the Rest and Digest challenge each day? If not – what was your roadblock?	
	start time	end time	total time fasted	check one	roadblock?
1. ____	to	____ hrs=		1. Yes__ No__	_____
2. ____	to	____ hrs=		2. Yes__ No__	_____
3. ____	to	____ hrs=		3. Yes__ No__	_____
4. ____	to	____ hrs=		4. Yes__ No__	_____
5. ____	to	____ hrs=		5. Yes__ No__	_____
6. ____	to	____ hrs=		6. Yes__ No__	_____
7. ____	to	____ hrs=		7. Yes__ No__	_____
8. ____	to	____ hrs=		8. Yes__ No__	_____
9. ____	to	____ hrs=		9. Yes__ No__	_____
10. ____	to	____ hrs=		10. Yes__ No__	_____
11. ____	to	____ hrs=		11. Yes__ No__	_____
12. ____	to	____ hrs=		12. Yes__ No__	_____
13. ____	to	____ hrs=		13. Yes__ No__	_____
14. ____	to	____ hrs=		14. Yes__ No__	_____

Notes _____

_____

_____

Ready, Set, Goal!

Rest and Digest
+ Refuel Time

Page 13   (For Daughter)

Record the time you stop eating when you begin to refuel. Take note of the total time fasted.

	start time	end time	total time fasted

1. ___ to ___ hrs=
2. ___ to ___ hrs=
3. ___ to ___ hrs=
4. ___ to ___ hrs=
5. ___ to ___ hrs=
6. ___ to ___ hrs=
7. ___ to ___ hrs=
8. ___ to ___ hrs=
9. ___ to ___ hrs=
10. ___ to ___ hrs=
11. ___ to ___ hrs=
12. ___ to ___ hrs=
13. ___ to ___ hrs=
14. ___ to ___ hrs=

Did you meet the Rest and Digest challenge each day? If not – what was your roadblock?

check one   roadblock?

1. Yes__ No__ _____
2. Yes__ No__ _____
3. Yes__ No__ _____
4. Yes__ No__ _____
5. Yes__ No__ _____
6. Yes__ No__ _____
7. Yes__ No__ _____
8. Yes__ No__ _____
9. Yes__ No__ _____
10. Yes__ No__ _____
11. Yes__ No__ _____
12. Yes__ No__ _____
13. Yes__ No__ _____
14. Yes__ No__ _____

Notes _____

Support & Report

To be done on Day 14:
It's time for show & tell!
Review your Goal Sheets together

Page 14

Accountability CTA (Call to Action)

This is a time for encouragement and reflection. You have tackled some important lifestyle changes in the past six weeks! Changes this significant can be hard! As you have learned the possibilities of finding freedom from sugar and highly processed food addictions, learned the importance of resting and digesting to give your body processes the healing and support they need to work as intended, you have been more intuitive of your body and its needs. If your goals include shedding fat and preventing disease, these strategies will get the job done. These are lifelong tools you will both use in supporting each other and sharing with your family as you continue on your journey.

It is now time to stop and reflect. How did it go? What did you find most challenging? Was there anything that surprised you? What is the most valuable thing you learned in Module #3? What is something you wish you had done differently? What are you most proud of? Take this time to collaborate. Write down your thoughts as you answer these prompts together. Get ready – your next module will open soon!

Notes

Sleep & Circadian Health

Aligning lifestyle with the body's natural daily rhythm for optimal health

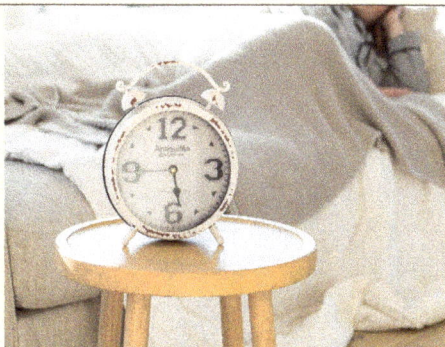

Welcome to Module #4. Your mother-daughter team is ready to learn the benefits of Circadian Health. Aligning with your circadian rhythm optimizes health by promoting better sleep, hormonal balance, and metabolism. It regulates appetite, aiding weight management, and enhances cognitive function.

Topics in this Module

- Understanding Circadian Rhythms
- Creating a Cirdian-Friendly Lifestyle
- Managing Light Exposure
- Tailoring Daily Habits

Synchronized circadian cycles contribute to improved mood, immune function, and overall well-being. Discovering and respecting your body's natural rhythm fosters lasting vitality, resilience, and a deeper connection to the innate balance of life. Together, you will learn to embrace circadian health for a harmonious approach to your overall health and well-being.

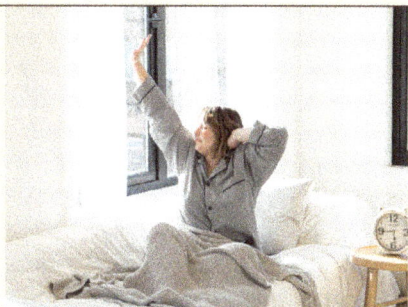

Notes

Time to Learn

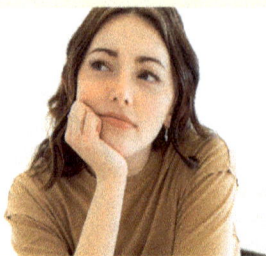

Page 1

Hello there, amazing wellness team! You are officially halfway through the EmpowHer modules! During the last 6 weeks, you have built a strong foundation for your new lifestyle. You have learned to value your body, prioritize protein, crowd out sugar, make healthy swaps, and time-restrict your eating window. As you move on to each new module, I encourage you to build upon the tools and habits learned every two weeks. By the time you finish all six modules, you will have the habits you need for your future health, mindset, food and body relationships, and weight management! Let's get started with Module #4!

What is a Circadian Rhythm?
Picture it as your body's built-in biological clock, governing a 24-hour cycle that repeats daily. It is not just a modern wellness buzzword – the concept dates back centuries. The term "circadian" itself stems from the Latin words "circa" (meaning 'around') and "diem" (meaning 'day'). It translates to "around a day."

Why Does it Matter?
Why should you care about this internal clock? Understanding and honoring your circadian rhythm comes with a multitude of perks. It is not just a health fad. It is about syncing with your body's natural flow to optimize your body's overall health.

Honoring Your Circadian Rhythm:
This is your natural 24-hour biological clock that regulates various physiological processes that can significantly contribute to weight loss for both younger and older women. The circadian rhythm influences essential functions such as sleep-wake cycles, hormone release, and metabolism. Adhering to these natural patterns can positively impact weight management through several mechanisms.

Notes _____

_____

_____

Time to Learn ☀

For Younger Women:
Respecting circadian rhythms is crucial for optimizing metabolism and energy expenditure. The body's internal clock dictates peak metabolic activity during the day, allowing for more efficient calorie burning. Aligning meals with the body's natural circadian cues, such as having a substantial breakfast while prioritizing protein and a lighter dinner, supports metabolic efficiency. Adequate sleep, another circadian-regulated factor, is essential as it affects hunger hormones—lack of sleep disrupts these hormones, increasing cravings for high-calorie foods.

For Older Women:
Hormonal changes, particularly during menopause, can affect weight distribution. Honoring the circadian rhythm becomes even more critical in this phase of life. Properly timed meals, time-restricted eating and regular sleep patterns contribute to hormone balance, mitigating factors that can lead to weight gain, insulin resistance, and cortisol fluctuations. Consistent sleep-wake cycles also play a role in preserving muscle mass, which is vital for maintaining a healthy weight as women age.

Adhering to circadian rhythms positively impacts psychological well-being. Stable sleep patterns and exposure to natural light during the day can reduce stress and emotional eating, promoting a healthier relationship with food. Respecting circadian rhythms aids weight loss in younger and older women by optimizing metabolism, regulating hormones, and supporting overall well-being. This approach acknowledges the interconnectedness of sleep, nutrition, and hormonal balance, providing a sustainable foundation for achieving and maintaining a healthy weight throughout different life stages.

Notes

Time to Learn

Rise and Shine!

Exposure to morning sunlight (particularly the blue wavelengths) stimulates the production of serotonin in the brain. It is beneficial to go outside, without sunglasses on, for 5-10 minutes in the morning. Expose yourself to wholesome Vitamin D! This practice also stimulates serotonin production. Serotonin is a neurotransmitter associated with mood regulation and wakefulness. Additionally, exposure to natural light helps regulate the body's internal circadian rhythm, influencing the release of melatonin, a crucial hormone in sleep-wake cycles.

When sunlight enters the eyes, it triggers a signal to the brain's suprachiasmatic nucleus (SCN), the internal clock that regulates circadian rhythms. This signal suppresses the production of melatonin, promoting alertness and signaling that it is time to be awake. This process not only helps synchronize the body's internal clock with the external day-night cycle but also contributes to overall well-being and mental alertness during the day.

Optimize Your Exercise Preferences
Morning or Afternoon: What Works Best For You?

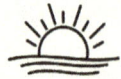

The circadian rhythm has a significant impact on various physiological processes, including exercise performance and recovery. Optimizing exercise with the circadian rhythm involves understanding how the body's natural fluctuations in temperature, hormone levels, and alertness can influence different aspects of physical activity.

Body Temperature Regulation:

The circadian rhythm influences core body temperature, which tends to be at its lowest in the early morning and highest in the late afternoon. Research suggests that body temperature elevation is associated with improved exercise performance. Therefore, exercising during the late afternoon or early evening may coincide with the body's peak temperature, potentially enhancing strength and endurance. Remember that when the sun begins its descent, your body should also start to wind down for optimal sleep.

Notes _____

_____

_____

Time to Learn

Hormonal Fluctuations:
Hormones like cortisol, associated with alertness and stress response, follow a circadian pattern. Cortisol levels typically peak in the early morning, providing a natural energy boost. Planning workouts during this time can take advantage of the increased cortisol levels, potentially leading to improved exercise performance. Choose what works best for your work, school, and social schedule. However, be aware of your circadian clock and hormone levels to make the most informed decision.

Muscle Strength and Coordination:
Studies have shown that muscle strength and coordination may be optimized in the afternoon. This may be attributed to factors such as increased body temperature, improved neural function, and enhanced muscle function during this time. Therefore, scheduling strength training or high-intensity workouts in the late afternoon might yield better results.

Recovery and Sleep:
Consistent exercise at the same time each day can help reinforce the body's circadian rhythm, potentially improving sleep quality. Quality sleep is crucial for recovery, muscle repair, and overall well-being, which are essential components of an effective exercise routine.

Aligning exercise with the circadian rhythm can enhance performance and optimize results. Factors such as body temperature, hormonal fluctuations, and the body's natural alertness levels should be considered when planning the timing of workouts. However, individual preferences, lifestyle, and commitments also play a role, so finding a consistent exercise routine that suits personal preferences and goals is key.

Notes _____

_____

_____

SLEEP DEPRIVATION
What happens?

10 DETRIMENTAL PROCESSES THAT OCCUR

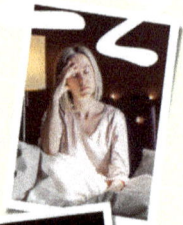

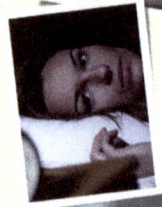

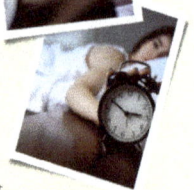

Insulin Resistance:
- Sleep deprivation can lead to insulin resistance. The body's cells become less responsive to insulin which results in elevated blood sugar levels.

Impaired Emotional Regulation:
- Insufficient sleep can impair the brain's ability to regulate emotions, making individuals more prone to irritability, mood swings, and heightened emotional reactivity.

Increased Cortisol Levels:
- Lack of sleep can lead to elevated cortisol levels. Increased cortisol can promote insulin resistance and stimulate the liver to produce more glucose, raising blood sugar levels.

Elevated Nighttime Glucose Levels:
- Sleep deprivation may contribute to elevated glucose levels during the night, disrupting the normal circadian rhythm of blood sugar regulation.

Altered Beta-Cell Function:
- Beta cells in the pancreas, responsible for insulin production, may not function optimally with insufficient sleep, leading to inadequate insulin secretion.

Increased Appetite and Cravings:
- Sleep deprivation can lead to changes in hormones that regulate hunger (ghrelin) and satiety (leptin), increasing appetite and cravings for high-carbohydrate and sugary foods.

Promotion of Inflammation:
- Chronic inflammation is associated with insulin resistance. Sleep deprivation can contribute to inflammation, further impacting insulin sensitivity.

Changes in Growth Hormone Release:
- Growth hormone, which plays a role in glucose metabolism, is released during deep sleep. Sleep deprivation can disrupt this release, affecting glucose regulation. Without human growth hormone, your body will miss out on the opportunity to build or maintain muscle.

Increased Risk of Type 2 Diabetes:
- Chronic sleep deprivation has been linked to an increased risk of developing type 2 diabetes due to its negative impact on insulin sensitivity and glucose metabolism.

Cognitive Impairment:
- Sleep deprivation affects cognitive functions such as memory, attention, and decision-making. It can lead to decreased alertness, difficulty concentrating, and impaired problem-solving.

Notes _____

_____

_____

GOOD SLEEP *What happens?*

The **glymphatic system** is a recently discovered waste clearance system in the brain, primarily active during sleep. This system facilitates the removal of waste products, including toxins and byproducts of neural activity, from the brain. During sleep, the space between brain cells expands, allowing cerebrospinal fluid to flow more efficiently, flushing out accumulated waste. This process supports overall brain health and function. Now, let's explore 10 additional benefits of getting good sleep:

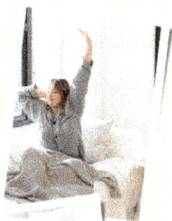

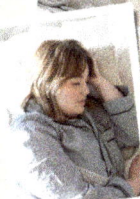

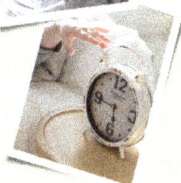

Weight Management:
- Sleep influences hormones that regulate hunger (ghrelin) and satiety (leptin). Adequate sleep helps maintain a healthy balance, supporting weight management and reducing the risk of obesity.

Blood Sugar Regulation:
- Quality sleep plays a role in insulin sensitivity and glucose metabolism. It helps regulate blood sugar levels, reducing the risk of insulin resistance and type 2 diabetes. This process supports unlocking fat stores.

Heart Health:
- A good night's sleep is associated with lower blood pressure and reduced stress on the cardiovascular system, reducing the risk of heart disease and stroke.

Enhanced Skin Health:
- Skin cells regenerate and repair during sleep. Adequate rest contributes to a healthier complexion, reduces the signs of aging, and supports overall skin health.

Stress Reduction:
- Sleep is a natural stress reliever. It helps regulate the stress hormone cortisol, promoting a sense of calm and aiding in stress management.

Cognitive Function:
- Adequate sleep is crucial for cognitive processes such as memory consolidation, learning, and problem-solving. It enhances attention, creativity, and decision-making.

Emotional Well-being:
- Quality sleep contributes to emotional resilience and stability. It helps regulate mood and decreases the likelihood of mood disorders like depression and anxiety.

Balances and Supports Hormone Function:
- Growth hormone, which plays a role in glucose metabolism, is released during deep sleep. Quality sleep can support this release, affecting glucose regulation.

Physical Recovery:
- During sleep, the body undergoes repair and restoration processes, promoting muscle growth, tissue repair, and the release of growth hormone. This is essential for overall physical well-being.

Immune System Support:
- Sleep is integral to a well-functioning immune system. It helps the body produce cytokines and antibodies, enhancing the ability to fight off infections and illnesses.

Notes

HOW TO PREPARE FOR
Good Sleep!

Honoring your circadian rhythm involves using science-based strategies to optimize various aspects of health and well-being, including sleep quality. Here are 10 science-backed methods for optimizing sleep:

Establish a Consistent Sleep Schedule:
- Going to bed and waking up at the same time every day, even on weekends, helps regulate your body's internal clock, promoting better sleep quality.

Create a Relaxing Bedtime Routine:
- Engage in calming activities before bedtime, such as reading, gentle stretching, or practicing relaxation techniques like deep breathing. This signals to your body that it's time to wind down.

Optimize Your Sleep Environment:
- Keep your bedroom cool, dark, and quiet. Invest in a comfortable mattress and pillows, and consider using blackout curtains to block out external light.

Limit Exposure to Screens Before Bed:
- The blue light emitted by screens can interfere with the production of melatonin, a hormone that regulates sleep. Limit screen time at least an hour before bedtime.

Mindfulness Meditation:
- Practicing mindfulness meditation has been shown to reduce stress and improve sleep quality. Techniques such as mindful breathing can help calm the mind before sleep.

Control Light Exposure:
- Expose yourself to natural light during the day, especially in the morning, to regulate your circadian rhythm. In the evening, reduce exposure to bright lights, and consider using dim, warm-colored lights.

Avoid Stimulants and Heavy Meals Before Bed:
- Caffeine and nicotine are stimulants that can interfere with sleep. Additionally, avoid heavy meals close to bedtime, as they may cause discomfort and disrupt sleep.

Exercise Regularly:
- Regular physical activity is associated with improved sleep quality. Aim for at least 30 minutes of moderate exercise most days of the week, but avoid vigorous workouts close to bedtime.

Consider Sleep Natural Supplements & Blue Light Blocking Glasses:
- Certain supplements, such as melatonin or magnesium, may help improve sleep quality for some individuals. Consult with a healthcare professional before incorporating supplements into your routine. Wear a good quality pair of blue light-blocking glasses to wear during screen time.

Use Sleep Tracking Technology:
- Wearable devices or smartphone apps that track your sleep patterns can provide insights into your sleep habits. This information can help you make adjustments to improve sleep quality.

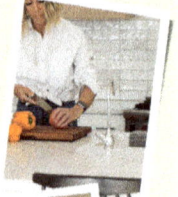

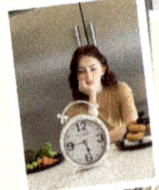

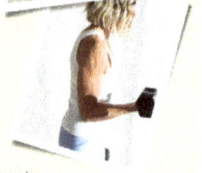

Notes _____

_____

_____

Pen to Paper
It's time to go to work!
Page 8

Daughter's Worksheet

Determine Your Chronotype:

Chronotypes are based on the idea that individuals have different natural preferences and peak times for various activities, influenced by their internal circadian rhythms. It's important to recognize that these are general categories, and individuals may not perfectly align with one specific chronotype.

1. What time do you naturally wake up on a day off?

a) Before 6 AM   b) Between 6 AM and 8 AM   c) After 8 AM

2. When do you feel most alert and productive during the day?

a) Early morning   b) Throughout the day   c) Evening and night

3. What is your preferred bedtime on a regular night?

a) Before 9 PM   b) Between 9 PM and 11 PM   c) After 11 PM

4. When do you usually have the most energy for physical activities or exercise?

a) Morning   b) Afternoon   c) Evening

5. How easily do you wake up in the morning?

a) Very easily   b) Moderately easily   c) Not easily

6. At what time do you find it most challenging to concentrate or stay focused?

a) Late morning   b) Afternoon   c) Evening

7. When do you tend to feel most relaxed and ready to unwind?

a) Evening   b) Consistently throughout the day   c) Morning

8. How do you feel about early morning commitments or obligations?

a) Preferable and energizing   b) Manageable but neutral   c) Challenging and draining

Notes _____

_____

_____

Pen to Paper
It's time to go to work!
Page 9

Mother's Worksheet

Determine Your Chronotype:

Chronotypes are based on the idea that individuals have different natural preferences and peak times for various activities, influenced by their internal circadian rhythms. It's important to recognize that these are general categories, and individuals may not perfectly align with one specific chronotype.

1. What time do you naturally wake up on a day off?

a) Before 6 AM   b) Between 6 AM and 8 AM   c) After 8 AM

2. When do you feel most alert and productive during the day?

a) Early morning   b) Throughout the day   c) Evening and night

3. What is your preferred bedtime on a regular night?

a) Before 9 PM   b) Between 9 PM and 11 PM   c) After 11 PM

4. When do you usually have the most energy for physical activities or exercise?

a) Morning   b) Afternoon   c) Evening

5. How easily do you wake up in the morning?

a) Very easily   b) Moderately easily   c) Not easily

6. At what time do you find it most challenging to concentrate or stay focused?

a) Late morning   b) Afternoon   c) Evening

7. When do you tend to feel most relaxed and ready to unwind?

a) Evening   b) Consistently throughout the day   c) Morning

8. How do you feel about early morning commitments or obligations?

a) Preferable and energizing   b) Manageable but neutral   c) Challenging and draining

Notes _____

_____

_____

Ready, Set, Goal!

It's time for some self-reflection & goal-setting!

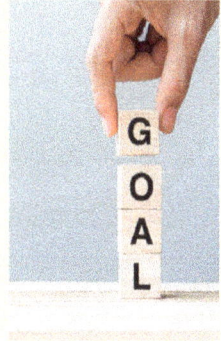

Page 10

Summary

There are several ways to categorize chronotypes, but one commonly used model identifies four main chronotypes. These are:

1. **Lion** (Mostly A's): Lions are early risers and tend to feel most alert and productive in the early morning. They naturally wake up early and may have a peak in energy and cognitive function during the first half of the day. Morning chronotypes typically prefer to schedule important tasks and activities in the morning.
2. **Bear** (Mostly B's): Bears have a balanced chronotype, experiencing relatively consistent energy levels and alertness throughout the day. They adapt well to different schedules and can function effectively at various times. Bears usually follow a sleep-wake pattern that aligns with the typical societal norms.
3. **Wolf** (Moslty C's): Wolves are evening chronotypes or "night owls." They prefer staying awake later into the night and may experience heightened alertness and productivity during the evening and nighttime hours. Wolves find it challenging to wake up early in the morning and may perform better during later parts of the day.
4. **Dolphin** (Mix of A's, B's and C's): Dolphins have irregular sleep patterns and may experience difficulties in maintaining a consistent sleep-wake cycle. They often have fragmented sleep and may find it challenging to adhere to conventional sleep schedules. Dolphins may not neatly fit into the traditional morning or evening chronotype categories.

These chronotypes are based on the idea that you have different natural preferences and peak times for various activities, influenced by your internal circadian rhythms. It is important to recognize that these are general categories that may give you insight into your individual sleep patterns. Whichever chronotype you fall into, prioritizing sleep is where you will find the most benefit with weight management and overall health.

Notes _____

_____

_____

Ready, Set, Goal!

Start a Bedtime Ritual to Optimize Sleep

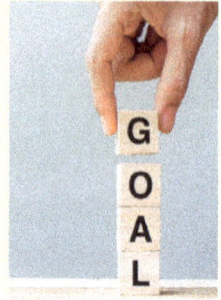

Page 11

You will both have a goal sheet that will require daily reflection and a record of your experience surrounding your sleep habits with recorded bedtimes. Keep the following information in mind when meeting these goals.

You will be asked to record your bedtime and wind-down habits along with your total hours of sleep. Here is why:

Recording sleep patterns fosters personal awareness. Tracking sleep duration, quality, and factors like bedtime routines pinpoint areas for improvement. Identifying patterns of poor sleep allows for targeted adjustments in your sleep hygiene.

Establishing consistent sleep routines and aligning daily activities with the body's internal rhythm not only improves sleep but also enhances overall health, including hormonal balance metabolic function, and weight management.

To wind down effectively for optimal sleep, prioritize dim lighting in the evening to signal to your body that it is time to rest. Gradually reduce screen time an hour or two before bed to limit exposure to artificial light. Wear blue light-blocking glasses if possible. Cut off your eating window at least two hours before bedtime, avoiding heavy or spicy meals that can disrupt digestion. Opt for calming activities such as reading, gentle stretching, or meditation. Avoid intense exercise close to bedtime, as it raises adrenaline levels.

Recording sleep habits is vital for optimizing sleep hygiene. Keeping a record of your sleep patterns helps you identify what is working and what is not. Track bedtime routines, screen time, and sleep duration. Identifying patterns can reveal connections between habits and sleep quality, guiding adjustments for better rest. This self-awareness empowers individuals to tailor their winding-down routine to suit their unique needs, fostering consistent and rejuvenating sleep.

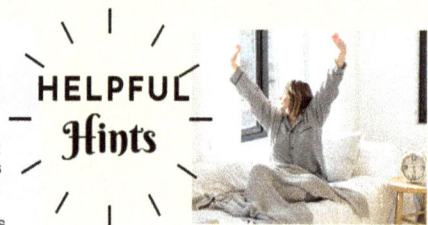

HELPFUL Hints

- Dim the lights and create more ambiance
- Limit screen time and artificial light
- Establish a relaxation ritual
- Engage in calming activities like reading
- Cut off your eating window
- Apply blue light filters to eyes or devices
- Keep your bedroom cool, dark and quiet
- Spend a few moments in gratitude & reflection
- Use the bathroom before bed
- Listen to a guided meditation app
- Move slow and speak softly
- Use a device to track sleep

Notes

Ready, Set, Goal!

Wake Up!

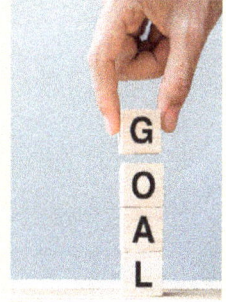

Page 12

As you support each other with good sleep hygiene habits, remember it takes time to figure out what is effective for you personally. Sleeping is a skill, and you will notice the benefits as you make it a priority. Be encouraged as you note these changes. Your body is learning to become more efficient and balanced. This process can take time. If you are paying attention, the results may surprise you!

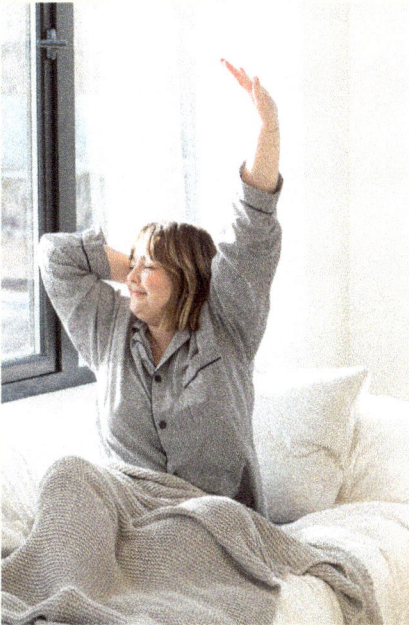

You will be asked to record your wake time and total hours slept. You will also determine your rituals to keep track of what is working or what is not. As you move forward, allow for different tactics. You will learn what best fits your needs according to your circadian rhythm. Meet this challenge each day and record any roadblocks and successes you encounter.

Waking up effectively sets the tone for the entire day, influencing peak performance, hormonal balance, and circadian rhythm synchronization. Exposure to natural light upon waking signals the body to suppress melatonin production, promoting alertness and aligning with the circadian rhythm. Engaging in morning rituals like stretching or a brief exercise session boosts endorphins, enhancing mood and energy levels.

Establishing a morning routine aids in regulating cortisol levels, the stress hormone, contributing to better stress management throughout the day. The synergy of these morning practices optimizes the body's hormonal balance, fostering sustained energy and mental clarity.

Recording progress is paramount in understanding the effectiveness of morning habits. Tracking wake-up time, energy levels, and adherence to routines provides valuable insights. Identifying patterns and tweaking habits based on recorded data helps refine morning rituals for continuous improvement. This approach to morning routines not only sets the foundation for peak performance but cultivates a proactive mindset, ensuring a more energized and focused start to each day.

Notes

Ready, Set, Goal!

Sleeping & Waking Rituals: Tracking for Circadian Health

Page 13   **For Mom**

Record the time you go to bed and when you rise in the morning. Take note of your total sleeping time.			Did you follow a sleep time and a wake time ritual? If "No" –what was your roadblock? If "Yes"– what worked?	
Bed time	Wake time	Total time sleeping	Check one	Roadblock or Success
1. ___ to ___	hrs=		1. Yes__ No__	___
2. ___ to ___	hrs=		2. Yes__ No__	___
3. ___ to ___	hrs=		3. Yes__ No__	___
4. ___ to ___	hrs=		4. Yes__ No__	___
5. ___ to ___	hrs=		5. Yes__ No__	___
6. ___ to ___	hrs=		6. Yes__ No__	___
7. ___ to ___	hrs=		7. Yes__ No__	___
8. ___ to ___	hrs=		8. Yes__ No__	___
9. ___ to ___	hrs=		9. Yes__ No__	___
10. ___ to ___	hrs=		10. Yes__ No__	___
11. ___ to ___	hrs=		11. Yes__ No__	___
12. ___ to ___	hrs=		12. Yes__ No__	___
13. ___ to ___	hrs=		13. Yes__ No__	___
14. ___ to ___	hrs=		14. Yes__ No__	___

Notes _____

_____

_____

Ready, Set, Goal!

Sleeping & Waking Rituals: Tracking for Circadian Health

For Daughter

Page 14

	Bed time	Wake time	Total time sleeping
Record the time you go to bed and when you rise in the morning. Take note of your total sleeping time.

1. ____ to ____ hrs=
2. ____ to ____ hrs=
3. ____ to ____ hrs=
4. ____ to ____ hrs=
5. ____ to ____ hrs=
6. ____ to ____ hrs=
7. ____ to ____ hrs=
8. ____ to ____ hrs=
9. ____ to ____ hrs=
10. ____ to ____ hrs=
11. ____ to ____ hrs=
12. ____ to ____ hrs=
13. ____ to ____ hrs=
14. ____ to ____ hrs=

Did you follow a sleep time and a wake time ritual? If "No" –what was your roadblock? If "Yes"– what worked?

Check one — Roadblock or Success

1. Yes__ No__ ____
2. Yes__ No__ ____
3. Yes__ No__ ____
4. Yes__ No__ ____
5. Yes__ No__ ____
6. Yes__ No__ ____
7. Yes__ No__ ____
8. Yes__ No__ ____
9. Yes__ No__ ____
10. Yes__ No__ ____
11. Yes__ No__ ____
12. Yes__ No__ ____
13. Yes__ No__ ____
14. Yes__ No__ ____

Notes ____

Support & Report

To be done on Day 14:
It's time for show & tell!
Review your Goal Sheets together

Page 15

Accountability CTA (Call to Action)

This is a time for encouragement and reflection. You have tackled some important lifestyle changes in the past eight weeks! Choices this significant require change. You have learned the possibilities of finding freedom from sugar and highly processed food addictions, learned the importance of resting and digesting to give your body processes the healing and support they need to work as intended, and have now tackled the importance of Circadian Health. You are on the right course if your goals include shedding fat, mood stability, hormone balance, and metabolic healing! These are lifelong tools you will use to support each other and share with your family as you continue your journey.

It is now time to stop and reflect. How did it go? What did you find most challenging? Was there anything that surprised you? What is the most valuable thing you learned in Module #4? What is something you wish you had done differently? What are you most proud of? Take this time to collaborate. Write down your thoughts as you answer these prompts together. Get ready –It is about time for your next module!

Notes

Module #5

Emotional vs Physical Hunger

Learning to establish the difference to optimize nutrition, a healthy mindset, and body

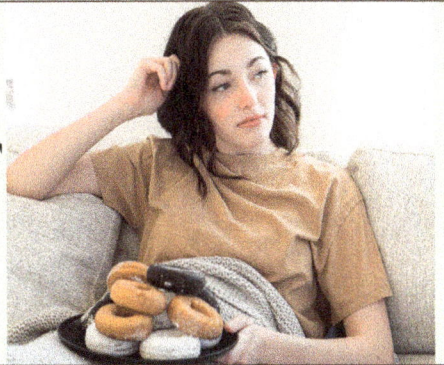

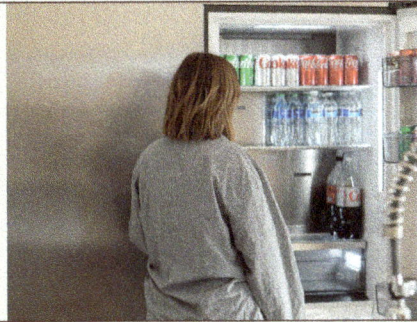

Welcome to Module #5! Your mother-daughter team is even closer to metabolic wellness! It is time to learn how to distinguish physical hunger cues from emotional triggers. Recognizing genuine hunger, while understanding emotional triggers fosters self-awareness. Encouraging mindful eating practices and promoting healthy coping mechanisms further empowers you to build a balanced relationship with food and emotions.

Topics in this Module

- Recognizing Physical Hunger
- Understand Emotional Hunger Triggers
- Mindful Eating Practices
- Healthy Coping Mechanisms

Understanding the distinctions between emotional, mental, and physical hunger is pivotal for optimal nutrition and overall well-being. Recognizing the unique cues of each hunger type enables you to make mindful dietary choices, fostering awareness of genuine nutritional needs. You can avoid impulsive or stress-induced eating by differentiating emotional cravings from physiological requirements. This heightened awareness contributes to healthier eating habits, supporting weight management and a balanced lifestyle. Emphasizing this approach empowers you to nourish your body and emotional and mental well-being, cultivating a sustainable foundation for lifelong health and vitality.

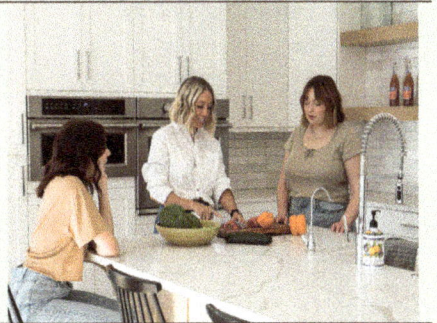

Notes _____

_____

_____

Time to Learn

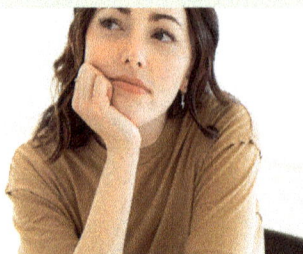

Page 1

The Process of Physcial Hunger:

Physical hunger is a complex physiological process regulated by hormones and the body's energy needs. When the body goes without food, it can efficiently switch fuel sources, utilizing both carbohydrates and fat for energy through a process called fat adaptation. This metabolic flexibility is essential for survival and occurs during prolonged periods without food. Often times we believe we are hungry because a certain amount of time has passed. If time is our only consideration, we are not allowing our body to use the fuel that is already present. This reveals the importance of recognizing actual physical hunger and intuition about when to refuel your body.

During the initial stages without food, the body depletes its glycogen stores, prompting the shift to fat metabolism. Fat cells release fatty acids, which are transported to the liver and converted into ketones, an alternative energy source. This adaptation allows the body to derive energy from stored fat efficiently.

Metabolic flexibility refers to the body's ability to switch between using carbohydrates and fat for fuel, reflecting a well-adapted and resilient metabolism. This flexibility is associated with improved insulin sensitivity and overall metabolic health.

After this adaptation, true physical hunger may arise. The body produces a hormone called ghrelin. It is characterized by stomach growling, a feeling of emptiness, or low energy levels. Distinguishing physical hunger from emotional hunger is crucial. Physical hunger develops gradually, allowing the body to adapt to a fasted state, while emotional hunger tends to be sudden and often triggered by stress, sleepiness or emotional cues.

To discern physical hunger, one can observe if the hunger persists and intensifies over time. Genuine hunger is also associated with an openness to various food options and is not specifically craving certain foods. Additionally, physical hunger is often satisfied by a balanced meal, whereas emotional hunger might persist even after eating. Understanding these scientific aspects aids in making informed decisions about nutritional intake, promoting a healthy relationship with food, and supporting overall well-being.

Notes _____

_____

_____

Time to Learn

The Process of Emotional Hunger:

This process is a phenomenon rooted in the intricate interplay of neurotransmitters and hormones within the brain. Stress, boredom, sadness, and other emotional triggers can prompt the brain to release neurotransmitters like serotonin and dopamine, influencing food cravings and emotional eating. Research indicates that emotional eating often involves the consumption of palatable, high-calorie foods, leading to weight gain.

The brain's reward centers, particularly the nucleus accumbens, play a role in associating certain foods with emotional comfort, contributing to the cycle of emotional eating. Chronic emotional eating can have detrimental effects on weight management, potentially leading to obesity and increased insulin resistance.

Insulin resistance, a condition where cells become less responsive to insulin, is linked to emotional eating patterns. Studies suggest that stress-induced emotional eating may contribute to insulin resistance, raising the risk of metabolic disorders.

Distinguishing emotional hunger from physical hunger is crucial. Emotional hunger tends to be sudden and often associated with specific cravings for comfort foods. Unlike physical hunger, emotional hunger may not be satisfied by a balanced meal and can persist even after overeating. Recognizing the emotional triggers and mindfully addressing emotional needs, such as stress reduction techniques, can help break the cycle of emotional eating.

Paying attention to the pace of eating and the types of foods desired can provide insights. Emotional hunger tends to lead to rapid consumption of specific comfort foods, while physical hunger develops gradually and is satisfied by a range of nutritious options. Understanding these neurobiological processes empowers you to make informed choices, promoting emotional well-being and facilitating healthier relationships with food.

Notes _____

_____

_____

Time to Learn

Eating When Physically Hungry:

This practice aligns with the body's natural signals, optimizing nutrient absorption and metabolic processes. When genuinely hungry, the digestive system is primed for efficient nutrient utilization, promoting energy balance and overall well-being. This approach supports metabolic flexibility, allowing the body to switch between fuel sources and maintain insulin sensitivity, contributing to long-term health benefits.

Eating When Emotionally Hungry:

Conversely, succumbing to emotional hunger, often driven by stress or boredom, can have detrimental effects. Emotional eating, particularly when indulging in highly palatable foods, triggers dopamine release in the brain, creating a reward response. Over time, this cycle can lead to an unhealthy dependence on emotional eating for comfort, resembling addictive patterns and contributing to weight gain and metabolic dysfunction.

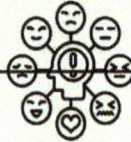

While there may be temporary emotional relief or comfort associated with succumbing to emotional hunger, it's important to note that these benefits are short-lived and come with potential long-term detriments. Emotional eating often involves consuming high-calorie, less nutritious foods, contributing to weight gain and associated health issues. The immediate psychological comfort may be overshadowed by negative impacts on overall well-being, including compromised physical health, increased risk of chronic diseases, and a potential reinforcing cycle of unhealthy eating patterns. Seeking alternative, healthier coping mechanisms for emotional distress is crucial for long-term emotional and physical health.

Notes

Time to Learn

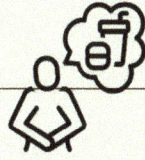

Physical Hunger Checklist:

☑️ **Gradual Onset:** Physical hunger tends to develop gradually. Assess if your hunger has built up over time rather than being sudden.

☑️ **Stomach Growling:** True physical hunger is often accompanied by stomach growling or rumbling. Pay attention to these physiological cues.

☑️ **Energy Levels:** Genuine hunger is associated with a decrease in energy levels and may make you feel fatigued or low on energy.

☑️ **Open to Various Foods:** Physical hunger is not specific to certain types of foods. If you're open to a variety of nutritious options, it may indicate genuine hunger.

☑️ **No Specific Cravings:** Unlike emotional hunger, which often involves cravings for specific comfort foods, physical hunger is not tied to particular cravings.

☑️ **Not Triggered by Emotional States:** Reflect on whether external factors like stress, boredom, or sadness triggered your hunger. True physical hunger is not emotionally driven.

☑️ **Hunger Persists:** Physical hunger tends to persist and intensify over time. If your hunger remains after eating, it may be more emotional than physical.

☑️ **Balanced Meal Satisfaction:** Physical hunger is typically satisfied by a balanced meal that includes a combination of proteins, fats, and carbohydrates.

☑️ **Mindful Eating:** Engage in mindful eating practices. Focus on the sensory experience of eating and listen to your body's signals of hunger and fullness.

☑️ **Hydration Check:** Sometimes, thirst can be mistaken for hunger. Ensure you are adequately hydrated before concluding hunger is physical.

Notes _____

_____

_____

Time to Learn

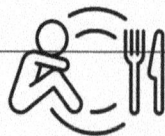

Emotional Hunger Checklist:

☑ **Sudden Onset:** Emotional hunger tends to be sudden and not related to a gradual buildup of physical hunger. Assess the immediacy of your hunger.

☑ **Specific Food Cravings:** Emotional hunger often involves cravings for specific comfort foods, especially those high in sugar, salt, or unhealthy fats.

☑ **Mindless Eating:** If you find yourself eating absentmindedly or without genuine hunger cues, it might be emotional eating rather than a physiological need.

☑ **Triggered by Emotions:** Reflect on whether your hunger is linked to emotional states such as stress, boredom, sadness, or anxiety.

☑ **Lack of Physical Hunger Signs**: Consider whether you are experiencing physical signs of hunger, such as stomach growling or low energy levels.

☑ **Eating Despite Fullness:** Emotional hunger may lead to overeating, even when physically full. Check if you continue eating despite no longer feeling hungry.

☑ **Comfort-Seeking Behavior:** Emotional hunger often arises from a desire for comfort or distraction. Assess if you are seeking solace through food.

☑ **Negative Emotions Post-Eating:** If feelings of guilt, regret, or sadness arise after eating, it may indicate that the hunger was emotionally driven.

☑ **Unsatisfying After Eating:** Emotional eating may not provide the satisfaction that comes with meeting genuine physical hunger. Evaluate whether your emotional needs are truly met by the food.

☑ **Pattern Recognition:** Reflect on any recurring patterns of emotional eating in specific situations or during particular emotional states.

Notes _____

_____

_____

Time to Learn

Once emotional hunger is determined, there are tools available that have been proven useful to deter the desire to eat emotionally. Together, as a mother-daugher team, you can support each other as you practice these options.

➤ **Try Mindfulness Meditation**: Engage in mindfulness meditation to increase awareness of emotional triggers and build resilience against impulsive eating, as supported by studies on mindfulness-based interventions.

➤ **Physical Activity**: Take a walk. Regular physical activity has been shown to reduce stress and improve mood by releasing endorphins, providing an effective alternative to emotional eating.

➤ **Journaling**: Scientific evidence supports the benefits of journaling in managing emotions. Write down feelings, thoughts, and triggers to gain clarity and develop healthier coping strategies.

➤ **Deep Breathing Exercises**: Deep breathing techniques activate the body's relaxation response, helping to alleviate stress and reduce the likelihood of turning to emotional eating.

➤ **Social Support**: Connect with friends, family, or part of your mother-daughter team. Positive social interactions release oxytocin, a hormone that counteracts stress and emotional eating tendencies.

➤ **Cognitive Behavioral Therapy (CBT)**: CBT has been proven effective in addressing emotional eating by identifying and modifying negative thought patterns and behaviors associated with food.

➤ **Healthy Food Choices:** Choose nutrient-dense foods that support mood and well-being. Certain foods, like those rich in protein with amino acids and healthy fat, have been linked to improved mental health.

➤ **Hydration**: Drinking water can help alleviate feelings of emptiness or cravings, and proper hydration is crucial for overall health and well-being. Drink a clean source of electrolytes to help with hydration.

➤ **Establishing Routine**: Creating a structured daily routine can provide a sense of control and stability, reducing the likelihood of succumbing to emotional eating triggers.

➤ **Seek Professional Guidance**: Consult with a registered dietitian, therapist, or counselor who can provide personalized strategies to manage emotional eating, based on evidence-based therapeutic approaches.

Notes

Pen to Paper

It's time to go to work!

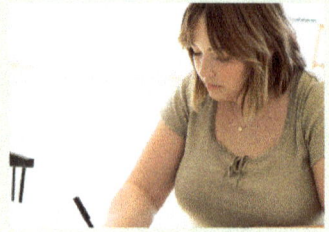

Daughter's Worksheet

What type of hungry are you really feeling?

Deciphering Hunger Cues – Emotional or Physical?

Rate each statement on a scale of 1 to 5, where 1 is strongly disagree, and 5 is strongly agree.

1. **I crave specific comfort foods when I feel hungry.**
   - (1) Strongly Disagree (2) Disagree (3) Neutral (4) Agree (5) Strongly Agree
2. **My hunger often arises suddenly and urgently.**
   - (1) Strongly Disagree (2) Disagree (3) Neutral (4) Agree (5) Strongly Agree
3. **I eat more when stressed, anxious, or sad.**
   - (1) Strongly Disagree (2) Disagree (3) Neutral (4) Agree (5) Strongly Agree
4. **I find myself snacking even when not physically hungry.**
   - (1) Strongly Disagree (2) Disagree (3) Neutral (4) Agree (5) Strongly Agree
5. **I often eat beyond the point of feeling full.**
   - (1) Strongly Disagree (2) Disagree (3) Neutral (4) Agree (5) Strongly Agree
6. **My hunger tends to be satisfied with a variety of foods.**
   - (1) Strongly Disagree (2) Disagree (3) Neutral (4) Agree (5) Strongly Agree
7. **I eat when bored, even if not hungry.**
   - (1) Strongly Disagree (2) Disagree (3) Neutral (4) Agree (5) Strongly Agree
8. **I often experience guilt or shame after eating.**
   - (1) Strongly Disagree (2) Disagree (3) Neutral (4) Agree (5) Strongly Agree
9. **I eat slowly and mindfully, savoring each bite.**
   - (1) Strongly Disagree (2) Disagree (3) Neutral (4) Agree (5) Strongly Agree
10. **I feel a physical sensation in my stomach when hungry.**
    - (1) Strongly Disagree (2) Disagree (3) Neutral (4) Agree (5) Strongly Agree

Notes _____

_____

_____

Pen to Paper

It's time to go to work!

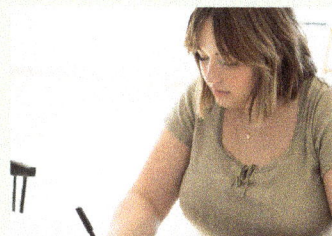

Page 8

Mom's Worksheet

What type of hungry are you really feeling?

Deciphering Hunger Cues – Emotional or Physical?

Rate each statement on a scale of 1 to 5, where 1 is strongly disagree, and 5 is strongly agree.

1. **I crave specific comfort foods when I feel hungry.**
   - (1) Strongly Disagree (2) Disagree (3) Neutral (4) Agree (5) Strongly Agree
2. **My hunger often arises suddenly and urgently.**
   - (1) Strongly Disagree (2) Disagree (3) Neutral (4) Agree (5) Strongly Agree
3. **I eat more when stressed, anxious, or sad.**
   - (1) Strongly Disagree (2) Disagree (3) Neutral (4) Agree (5) Strongly Agree
4. **I find myself snacking even when not physically hungry.**
   - (1) Strongly Disagree (2) Disagree (3) Neutral (4) Agree (5) Strongly Agree
5. **I often eat beyond the point of feeling full.**
   - (1) Strongly Disagree (2) Disagree (3) Neutral (4) Agree (5) Strongly Agree
6. **My hunger tends to be satisfied with a variety of foods.**
   - (1) Strongly Disagree (2) Disagree (3) Neutral (4) Agree (5) Strongly Agree
7. **I eat when bored, even if not hungry.**
   - (1) Strongly Disagree (2) Disagree (3) Neutral (4) Agree (5) Strongly Agree
8. **I often experience guilt or shame after eating.**
   - (1) Strongly Disagree (2) Disagree (3) Neutral (4) Agree (5) Strongly Agree
9. **I eat slowly and mindfully, savoring each bite.**
   - (1) Strongly Disagree (2) Disagree (3) Neutral (4) Agree (5) Strongly Agree
10. **I feel a physical sensation in my stomach when hungry.**
    - (1) Strongly Disagree (2) Disagree (3) Neutral (4) Agree (5) Strongly Agree

Notes _____

_____

_____

Ready, Set, Goal!

It's time for some self-reflection & goal-setting!

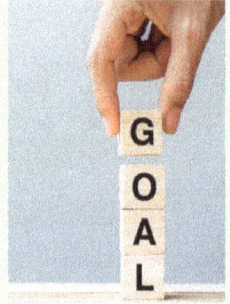

Page 9

Summary

Answer Key:
- Add up the scores for questions (Group E) 1, 3, 4, 7, and 8   Score=_____
- Add up the scores for questions (Group P) 2, 5, 6, 9, and 10   Score=_____

Interpretation:

Emotional Hunger (Group E) Total score 5-15: If your score falls in this range, it may suggest that your hunger cues are more influenced by emotional factors. High scores on questions related to specific cravings, eating in response to emotions, and feeling guilt after eating indicate a potential connection between your eating habits and emotional states.

Physical Hunger (Group P) Total score 20-25: A higher total score in this range may signify a stronger connection to physical hunger cues. Questions emphasizing the gradual onset of hunger, satisfaction with various foods, and the presence of physical sensations in the stomach point towards a more intuitive and body-driven approach to eating.
Possible Outcomes and Meanings:

- **Emotional Eater**: A tendency toward emotional eating can lead to eating for comfort or distraction rather than true physical hunger. Strategies like mindful eating, identifying emotional triggers, and finding alternative coping mechanisms may be beneficial.
- **Intuitive Eater:** A higher score on questions related to physical hunger suggests a better connection to the body's natural cues. Embracing mindful eating practices, focusing on hunger and fullness cues, and choosing a variety of nutrient-dense foods can contribute to a more balanced and intuitive approach to eating.

Remember, these scores offer insights and not definitive diagnoses. A combination of emotional and physical factors influences our eating habits, and adopting a mindful and intuitive approach to eating can contribute to a healthier relationship with food. Always consult with healthcare or nutrition professionals for personalized advice.

Notes _____

_____

_____

Ready, Set, Goal!

Prioritizing Protein

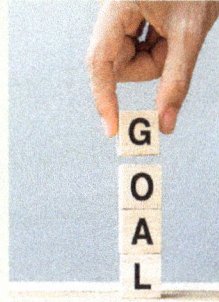

Page 10

You will both have a goal sheet that will require daily reflection and a record of your experience surrounding emotional and physical hunger. Keep the following information in mind when meeting these goals.

You will be asked to track "physical hunger cues." Here is why:

Tracking physical hunger cues is crucial for cultivating intuitive eating habits. By noting sensations like stomach growling, energy levels, and gradual hunger onset, individuals gain a deeper understanding of their body's needs. This awareness enables more mindful food choices aligned with genuine hunger, fostering a healthier relationship with eating. Regularly tracking physical hunger cues empowers individuals to distinguish between true hunger and emotional triggers, promoting a balanced and intuitive approach to nourishment.

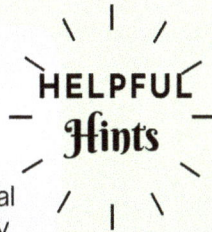

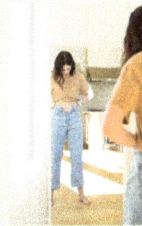

HELPFUL Hints

- Note stomach sensations like rumbling
- Observe dipping energy levels
- Observe a gradual onset rather than sudden
- Observe mood – less emotion with true hunger
- Ensure adequate hydration
- Pay attention to flavors and textures
- Ensure nutrient-dense foods and protein
- Aim to eat when hungry – not because it is time
- Listen to what a craving might be telling you
- Cultivate a strong mind–body connection
- Listen to your body without judgment
- Be curious and learn from your body's cues

Notes _____

Ready, Set, Goal!

Let's Swap!

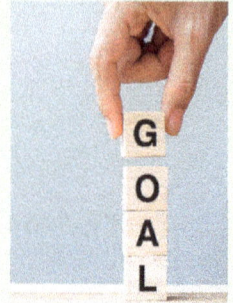

Page 11

As you support each other in deciphering the difference between physical and emotional hunger, it is important to remember to stay non-judgemental about each other's experience as well as your own body. Learning about the mind-body connection is a process, and you have made great strides in tuning in to the cues your body has given you. This is an important step in your lifestyle change. Listen to these cues as you meet your next goal.

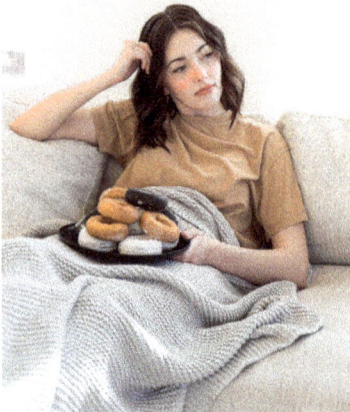

You will be asked to track "emotional hunger triggers." Here is why:

Tracking emotional hunger is vital for fostering a healthy relationship with food. Identifying specific triggers, such as stress, boredom, or sadness, allows individuals to recognize patterns and understand the emotional roots of their eating habits. This awareness empowers proactive, mindful responses rather than impulsive reactions to emotions through food. Once triggers are identified, developing alternative coping mechanisms, like deep breathing, journaling, or engaging in activities that bring joy, redirects emotional responses away from food. By tracking emotional hunger, individuals can break the cycle of using food as a primary emotional outlet, leading to more balanced and intuitive eating habits. Cultivating a healthy relationship with food and body.

Notes _____

_____

_____

Ready, Set, Goal!

Identifying physical and emotional hunger

Page 12   **For Mom**

Write down your physical hunger level 1-5 (less to great) when breaking your fast for the day. Next, track your satisfaction level 1-5 after fueling your body.		Did you notice any emotional hunger from day to day? If so, identify your triggers like boredom, sadness, anger, anxiety, etc. Then track the redirection skill you practiced.	
rate 1 – 5	rate 1 – 5	check one	trigger/redirect
1. _____	Satisfaction=	1. Yes__ No__	_____
2. _____	Satisfaction=	2. Yes__ No__	_____
3. _____	Satisfaction=	3. Yes__ No__	_____
4. _____	Satisfaction=	4. Yes__ No__	_____
5. _____	Satisfaction=	5. Yes__ No__	_____
6. _____	Satisfaction=	6. Yes__ No__	_____
7. _____	Satisfaction=	7. Yes__ No__	_____
8. _____	Satisfaction=	8. Yes__ No__	_____
9. _____	Satisfaction=	9. Yes__ No__	_____
10. _____	Satisfaction=	10. Yes__ No__	_____
11. _____	Satisfaction=	11. Yes__ No__	_____
12. _____	Satisfaction=	12. Yes__ No__	_____
13. _____	Satisfaction=	13. Yes__ No__	_____
14. _____	Satisfaction=	14. Yes__ No__	_____

Notes _____

_____

_____

Ready, Set, Goal!

For Daughter

Page 13

Identifying physical and emotional hunger

	rate 1 – 5	rate 1 – 5		check one	trigger/redirect
	Write down your physical hunger level 1-5 (less to great) when breaking your fast for the day. Next, track your satisfaction level 1–5 after fueling your body.			Did you notice any emotional hunger from day to day? If so, identify your triggers like boredom, sadness, anger, anxiety, etc. Then track the redirection skill you practiced.	
1	_____ Satisfaction=		1	Yes__ No__	_____
2.	_____ Satisfaction=		2.	Yes__ No__	_____
3.	_____ Satisfaction=		3.	Yes__ No__	_____
4.	_____ Satisfaction=		4.	Yes__ No__	_____
5.	_____ Satisfaction=		5.	Yes__ No__	_____
6.	_____ Satisfaction=		6.	Yes__ No__	_____
7.	_____ Satisfaction=		7.	Yes__ No__	_____
8.	_____ Satisfaction=		8.	Yes__ No__	_____
9.	_____ Satisfaction=		9.	Yes__ No__	_____
10.	_____ Satisfaction=		10.	Yes__ No__	_____
11	_____ Satisfaction=		11	Yes__ No__	_____
12.	_____ Satisfaction=		12.	Yes__ No__	_____
13.	_____ Satisfaction=		13.	Yes__ No__	_____
14.	_____ Satisfaction=		14.	Yes__ No__	_____

Notes _____

_____

_____

Support & Report

To be done on Day 14:
It's time for show & tell!
Review your Goal Sheets together

Page 14

Accountability CTA (Call to Action)

This is a time for celebration and reflection. You have made some important lifestyle changes these past two weeks. These changes give you a glimpse into your new health-driven lifestyle. You have uncovered future possibilities as you have learned specific health strategies throughout this course. Suppose your goals include body acceptance, body recomposition, insulin sensitivity, healing your metabolism for sustainable weight loss, finding value in circadian health, and learning to decipher emotional hunger. In that case, these are the lifelong tools you will both use in supporting each other and sharing with your family as you continue on your journey.

It is now time to stop and reflect. How did it go? What did you find most challenging? Was there anything that surprised you? What is the most valuable thing you learned in Module #5? What is something you wish you had done differently? What are you most proud of? Take this time to collaborate. Write down your thoughts as you answer these prompts together. Get ready - It is almost time to start your next module!

Notes

Metabolism & Muscle Health

Metabolic healing by supporting a muscle-centric lifestyle

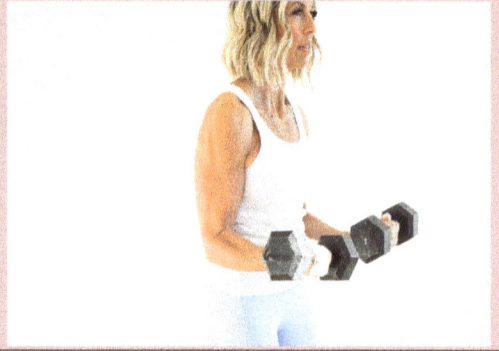

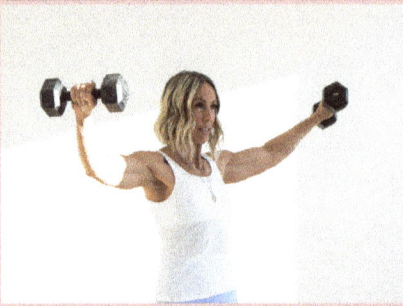

Welcome to Module #6! All six modules come together as you learn the magic of living a muscle-centric lifestyle and the profound health benefits it offers your mother-daughter team. Prioritizing a protein-forward diet and clean, nutrient-rich foods supports metabolic health, promoting sustained energy and weight. Engaging in exercise that stimulates healthy muscle growth not only enhances strength but also aids in disease prevention, fosters metabolic freedom, and contributes to overall weight management. This approach promotes a strong foundation for sustainable, long-term health.

Topics in this Module

- Explore a Muscle-Centric Lifestyle
- Understand a Muscle-Centric Diet
- Learn the role of Muscle-Centric Exercise
- Incorporate Mindset for Metabolic Health

Living a muscle-centric lifestyle is a powerful catalyst for metabolic health. A diet rich in protein and nutrients fuels the body's metabolic engine, supporting efficient calorie burning. Incorporating resistance training builds and maintains lean muscle mass, boosting metabolism and insulin sensitivity. The mindset completes the triad, fostering a holistic approach to well-being. By synergizing a nutrient-dense diet, purposeful exercise, and a positive mindset, individuals unlock sustained metabolic health, weight management, and well-being.

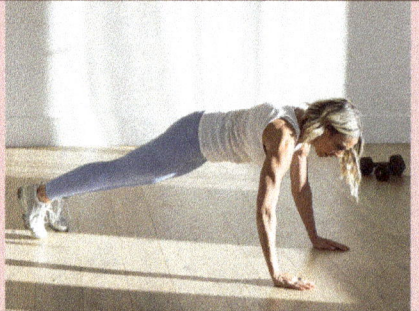

Notes _____

_____

_____

Time to Learn

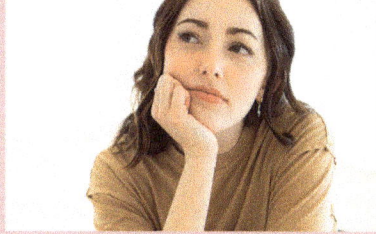

Page 1

Why is Muscle so Important?

The history of the muscle-centric lifestyle is rooted in evolutionary biology. Our ancestors, reliant on physical activity for survival, naturally maintained robust muscle mass. Today, sedentary lifestyles contribute to muscle loss, **a phenomenon more detrimental than fat gain**. Loss of muscle, termed sarcopenia, accelerates aging and triggers weight gain and metabolic diseases.

Muscle tissue is pivotal in glucose metabolism, insulin sensitivity, and energy expenditure. Muscle loss, or sarcopenia, plays a crucial role in metabolic diseases. Its decline is linked to obesity, diabetes, dementia, heart disease, PCOS, and Alzheimer's.

Beyond metabolic health, muscle-centric living is paramount for weight management. Muscle tissue is metabolically active, burning calories at rest and supporting a healthy body composition. In contrast, the loss of muscle diminishes this calorie-burning capacity, making weight management challenging.

Eating a protein-forward diet to support muscle health and adding resistance training are integral to a muscle-centric lifestyle, not only combat muscle loss but to enhance metabolic health and effective weight management. Embracing this lifestyle is a healthy approach to preventing and managing a spectrum of metabolic diseases while supporting sustainable weight management.

Notes _____

_____

_____

Time to Learn

A Muscle-Centric Diet:

Prioritize a protein-forward approach to support muscle health and overall well-being. Include lean protein sources such as poultry, fish, quality meats, dairy, and eggs. Protein is essential for muscle repair, growth, and overall metabolic health.

A protein-forward diet offers numerous benefits. Firstly, protein has a high thermic effect of food (TEF), meaning the body expends more energy to digest and process it compared to fats or carbohydrates. This elevates the overall calorie expenditure, contributing to weight management and metabolic efficiency. Additionally, protein-rich meals induce a feeling of satiety, reducing overall calorie intake and supporting weight control.

Muscle protein synthesis (MPS) is a crucial process in building and repairing muscle tissue. It involves the incorporation of amino acids, the building blocks of proteins, into muscle fibers. Consuming an adequate amount of high-quality protein, especially those rich in essential amino acids, stimulates MPS. Branched-chain amino acids (BCAAs), like leucine, play a particularly significant role in this process. Regular protein intake, enhances MPS, promoting muscle strength, recovery, and overall metabolic health.

Adopting a muscle-centric diet involves prioritizing high-quality protein sources, harnessing the thermic effect of food, and understanding the nuances of muscle protein synthesis. This dietary approach not only supports muscle health but also contributes to weight management and metabolic efficiency.

> Refer to Module #2 to brush up on prioritizing protein. Page 10 offers some "Helpful Hints" to encourage hitting your protein goals each day as you now understand the importance of muscle protein synthesis (MPS). The latest research suggests the optimal amount of protein daily to be at least one gram of protein per desired body weight. If you desire to be the size of a 140 lb person, you should aim for 140 grams of protein.

Notes _____

_____

_____

Time to Learn

Muscle-Centric Exercise:

- Prioritizing muscle gain over excessive cardio involves understanding the profound impact of resistance training and a high-protein diet on metabolism, disease prevention, body composition, metabolic flexibility, and weight management.

- Resistance training, a hallmark of muscle-centric living, triggers muscle protein synthesis (MPS), contributing to muscle growth. Unlike cardio, which primarily burns calories during exercise, increased muscle mass elevates resting metabolic rate, promoting continuous calorie burning. This metabolic boost is crucial for maintaining a healthy weight and fostering metabolic flexibility, allowing the body to efficiently switch between energy sources.

- Focusing on muscle gain has protective effects against metabolic diseases. Muscle is a key player in glucose metabolism, enhancing insulin sensitivity and reducing the risk of metabolic diseases. Additionally, resistance training positively influences lipid profiles, lowering the risk of cardiovascular diseases.

- Prioritizing muscle gain through resistance training and a high-protein diet offers a pathway toward desired body composition. Muscle enhances your confidence, strength in daily tasks, and overall appearance. Muscle not only protects but accomplishes the desired aesthetic most women are searching for.

Notes _____
_____
_____

Time to Learn

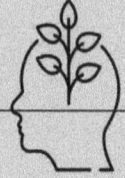

Incorporating a Positive Muscle-Centric Mindset:
This is a crucial element when striving for metabolic health within a muscle-centric lifestyle. Cultivating a mindset that aligns with your health goals enhances adherence to dietary and exercise habits.

1. **Set Realistic Goals:**
   - Begin with achievable and realistic goals that are specific, measurable, and time-bound. Celebrate small victories, fostering a positive mindset and motivation for sustained efforts.

2. **Embrace the Process:**
   - Shift focus from immediate outcomes to appreciating the journey. Understand that metabolic health and muscle gain are gradual processes requiring consistency. Develop a mindset that values this process and the time it takes to become metabolically well.

3. **Practice Mindful Eating:**
   - Approach meals with mindfulness, savoring the flavors and nourishing your body. A positive mindset around food reduces stress and emotional eating, contributing to overall metabolic health.

4. **View Exercise as Self-Care:**
   - Frame exercise as a form of self-care rather than a chore. Understand that each workout contributes to your well-being, both mentally and physically. Enjoying a healthy, active body is a privilege, not a punishment. Keep this in mind when practicing muscle-centric exercise.

5. **Celebrate Non-Scale Victories:**
   - Go beyond the scale. Celebrate non-scale victories such as increased energy levels, improved mood, enhanced strength, and change in body composition. Gaining muscle and losing fat does NOT show up on a scale! A positive mindset recognizes metabolic health beyond numerical metrics.

6. **Cultivate Resilience:**
   - View setbacks as opportunities for discoveries about your body rather than failures. Cultivate resilience by learning from challenges and adapting your approach. A resilient mindset contributes to long-term success.

7. **Practice Gratitude:**
   - Express gratitude for your body's abilities and the ability to pursue a muscle-centric lifestyle that will bring you sustainable health and disease prevention. A grateful mindset reinforces a positive relationship with your body and your journey toward metabolic health.

Notes _____

_____

_____

Time to Learn

how it all connects

The integration of these six modules creates the framework for achieving sustainable metabolic health, disease prevention, and effective body fat management. Scientifically grounded principles guide the synergy between these topics, highlighting their interdependence and cumulative impact on overall health.

1. **Sugar Crowding and Body Confidence:**
   - Reducing sugar intake aligns with the principles of a circadian health approach, influencing sleep quality and optimizing metabolic function. Scientific studies, such as those in the Journal of Clinical Sleep Medicine, emphasize the bidirectional relationship between sleep and metabolic health. Improved sleep supports hormonal balance, fostering body confidence as individuals experience enhanced energy levels and reduced stress, positively impacting body image.

2. **Processed Foods and Seed Oils:**
   - Eliminating highly processed foods and seed oils aligns with the muscle-centric lifestyle by providing nutrient-dense, anti-inflammatory foods. Research in the American Journal of Clinical Nutrition emphasizes the impact of anti-inflammatory diets on metabolic health. As we prioritize protein-rich, whole foods, we support muscle growth and create an environment that discourages inflammation, a crucial aspect of disease prevention.

3. **Protein Prioritization:**
   - Prioritizing protein complements the circadian health module by considering the timing of protein intake. Scientific literature, including studies in the American Journal of Physiology, highlights the importance of protein distribution throughout the day for muscle protein synthesis and metabolic health. Adequate protein intake also supports satiety, linking to the module on recognizing physical versus emotional hunger.

4. **Circadian Health and Time-Restricted Eating:**
   - Circadian health and the importance of sleep are foundational to all modules. The Journal of Clinical Endocrinology & Metabolism illustrates the impact of disrupted circadian rhythms on metabolism. Prioritizing sleep influences hormonal regulation, contributing to effective muscle recovery and fat metabolism. Time-restricted eating extends to circadian health and sleep. This way of eating also supports intuitive eating and an understanding of hunger cues while lowering blood sugar and insulin to support testosterone and HGH (human growth hormone), which supports a muscle-centric lifestyle and metabolic health.

5. **Understanding Hunger:**
   - Distinguishing between physical and emotional hunger ties back to circadian health and muscle-centric living. Scientific evidence in the American Journal of Clinical Nutrition emphasizes the role of protein in satiety and appetite regulation. A muscle-centric lifestyle and balanced circadian rhythms promote a healthier relationship with food.

6. **Muscle-Centric Living:**
   - Leading a muscle-centric lifestyle integrates all modules by actively contributing to disease prevention, metabolic health, and effective body fat management. Research in the International Journal of Obesity highlights the role of resistance training in improving body composition and metabolic parameters.

These modules form a cohesive narrative that addresses metabolic health from multiple angles. By acknowledging the interconnectedness of sugar reduction, whole food choices, protein prioritization, time-restricted eating, circadian health, hunger awareness, and muscle-centric living, you can cultivate a sustainable approach to health, fostering disease prevention and effective body weight and muscle management.

Notes

Time to Learn

Muscle Is the Organ Of Metabolic Health:

A three-day resistance training routine can be effective for beginners aiming to enhance body composition and gain muscle in the weight room (or at home). Remember to start light until you get the correct form. **With the help of a trainer or someone more experienced**, feel free to add more exercises and workout days and increase weight to optimize muscle building. It doesn't need to be complicated. Here is a simple way to get started. If you do not see resistance training in your future - find something that puts a demand on your skeletal muscle system and do it! While individual activity needs may vary, accumulating approximately 10,000 steps daily has been associated with various health benefits, including improved cardiovascular and metabolic health. If you are starting from ground zero (the couch), take it easy, but get moving to optimize the healthy habits you have implemented in the last ten weeks.

Upper Body Day: (day 1 – Monday)

Perform compound exercises such as bench press, overhead press, and bent-over rows. Aim for 3 sets of 8–12 repetitions for each exercise. Focus on controlled movements, emphasizing the eccentric (lowering) phase. You eventually will want to work to "muscle failure" at around 12-15 reps. If you are not to that point - start to add more weight.

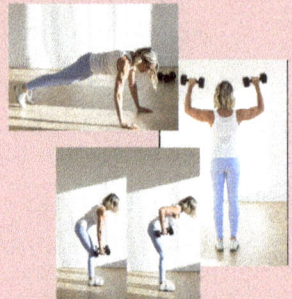

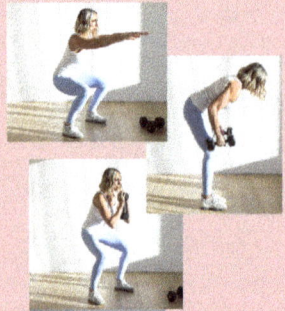

Lower Body Day: (day 2 – Wednesday)

Include squats, deadlifts, and lunges as foundational exercises. Execute 3 sets of 8-12 reps per exercise, gradually increasing weight as strength improves. Prioritize proper form to prevent injury and optimize muscle engagement. You eventually will want to work to "muscle failure" at around 12-15 reps. If you are not to that point - start to add more weight.

Full Body Day: (day 3 – Friday)

Combine compound movements like deadlifts, squats, overhead press, and push-ups. Incorporate 3-4 sets of 8-12 reps for each exercise. This full-body approach ensures comprehensive muscle activation and an efficient use of training time.

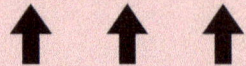

Notes _____

_____

_____

Pen to Paper

It's time to go to work!

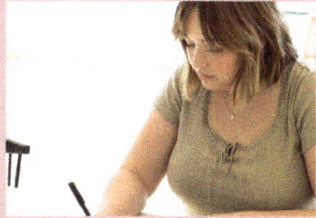

Page 7

Daughter's Worksheet: Part 1

Look at all you have
learned and practiced

Let's see how you are doing and determine where we can celebrate and where we can adjust.
Rate each statement on a scale of 1 to 5, where 1 is strongly disagree, and 5 is strongly agree.

1. I have cut out sugar and benefit from fewer energy crashes, cravings, and mood swings.
(1)Strongly Disagree (2) Disagree (3) Neutral (4) Agree (5) Strongly Agree

2. I've learned to appreciate my body and have positive thoughts and actions toward it.
(1) Strongly Disagree (2) Disagree (3) Neutral (4) Agree (5) Strongly Agree

3. I have prioritized quality protein and eat at least 30 grams per meal.
(1) Strongly Disagree (2) Disagree (3) Neutral (4) Agree (5) Strongly Agree

4. I understand which seed oils to avoid and what healthy alternatives are to replace them.
(1) Strongly Disagree (2) Disagree (3) Neutral (4) Agree (5) Strongly Agree

5. I follow my circadian rhythm and find it important to rest and digest as I practice time-restricted eating.
(1) Strongly Disagree (2) Disagree (3) Neutral (4) Agree (5) Strongly Agree

6. I understand the benefits of time-restricted eating and fueling my body during my eating window.
(1) Strongly Disagree (2) Disagree (3) Neutral (4) Agree (5) Strongly Agree

7. I make it a priority to get quality sleep and hit 7-8 hours nightly.
(1) Strongly Disagree (2) Disagree (3) Neutral (4) Agree (5) Strongly Agree

8. I practice a ritual that helps me prepare for quality sleep.
(1) Strongly Disagree (2) Disagree (3) Neutral (4) Agree (5) Strongly Agree

9. I listen to hunger cues and can decipher when I feel emotional or physical hunger.
(1) Strongly Disagree (2) Disagree (3) Neutral (4) Agree (5) Strongly Agree

Notes _____

_____

_____

Pen to Paper

It's time to go to work!

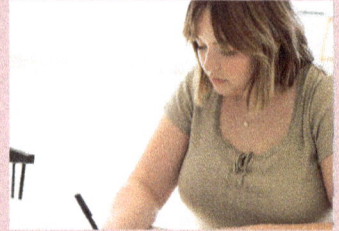

Page 8

Daughter's Worksheet: Part 2

10. When I determine I feel emotional hunger, I practice redirecting skills and avoid the temptation to eat when I am not physically hungry.

(1) Strongly Disagree (2) Disagree (3) Neutral (4) Agree (5) Strongly Agree

11. I understand the important role muscle plays in my metabolic health.

(1) Strongly Disagree (2) Disagree (3) Neutral (4) Agree (5) Strongly Agree

12. I understand that by leaning into this mindset, I can enjoy weight management and disease prevention.

(1) Strongly Disagree (2) Disagree (3) Neutral (4) Agree (5) Strongly Agree

As you reflect on your self-assessment, celebrate your achievements and acknowledge areas for personal growth. High ratings in body appreciation and cutting out sugar signify a positive relationship with yourself and a commitment to reducing potential health risks. Similarly, crowding out highly processed foods demonstrates a dedication to nourishing your body with wholesome options, fostering overall weight management and mental health.

A high rating in time-restricted eating practices aligns with metabolic health, emphasizing the importance of optimal digestion and autophagy and lowered insulin levels. Prioritizing sleep and aligning with your circadian rhythm is crucial for hormonal balance and overall health. Recognizing and responding to physical rather than emotional hunger showcases mindfulness, contributing to a healthy relationship with food.

View those areas with lower ratings as opportunities for personal adjustments. Identify actionable steps to enhance these aspects of your lifestyle, supporting your transformation toward sustainable metabolic health and overall well-being. Your journey is dynamic, and these self-reflections provide a roadmap for continuous growth and positive lifestyle changes.

Notes _____

_____

_____

Pen to Paper

It's time to go to work!

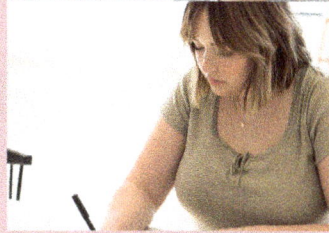

Mother's Worksheet: Part 1

Look at all you have
learned and practiced

Let's see how you are doing and determine where we can celebrate and where we can adjust.
Rate each statement on a scale of 1 to 5, where 1 is strongly disagree, and 5 is strongly agree.

1. I have cut out sugar and benefit from fewer energy crashes, cravings, and mood swings.
(1)Strongly Disagree (2) Disagree (3) Neutral (4) Agree (5) Strongly Agree

2. I've learned to appreciate my body and have positive thoughts and actions toward it.
(1) Strongly Disagree (2) Disagree (3) Neutral (4) Agree (5) Strongly Agree

3. I have prioritized quality protein and eat at least 30 grams per meal.
(1) Strongly Disagree (2) Disagree (3) Neutral (4) Agree (5) Strongly Agree

4. I understand which seed oils to avoid and what healthy alternatives are to replace them.
(1) Strongly Disagree (2) Disagree (3) Neutral (4) Agree (5) Strongly Agree

5. I follow my circadian rhythm and find it important to rest and digest as I practice time-restricted eating.
(1) Strongly Disagree (2) Disagree (3) Neutral (4) Agree (5) Strongly Agree

6. I understand the benefits of time-restricted eating and fueling my body during my eating window.
(1) Strongly Disagree (2) Disagree (3) Neutral (4) Agree (5) Strongly Agree

7. I make it a priority to get quality sleep and hit 7-8 hours nightly.
(1) Strongly Disagree (2) Disagree (3) Neutral (4) Agree (5) Strongly Agree

8. I practice a ritual that helps me prepare for quality sleep.
(1) Strongly Disagree (2) Disagree (3) Neutral (4) Agree (5) Strongly Agree

9. I listen to hunger cues and can decipher when I feel emotional or physical hunger.
(1) Strongly Disagree (2) Disagree (3) Neutral (4) Agree (5) Strongly Agree

Notes _____

_____

_____

Pen to Paper

It's time to go to work!

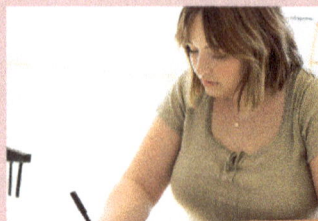

Mother's Worksheet: Part 2

10. When I determine I feel emotional hunger, I practice redirecting skills and can avoid the temptation to eat when I am not physically hungry.
(1) Strongly Disagree (2) Disagree (3) Neutral (4) Agree (5) Strongly Agree

11. I understand the important role muscle plays in my metabolic health.
(1) Strongly Disagree (2) Disagree (3) Neutral (4) Agree (5) Strongly Agree

12. I understand that by leaning into this mindset, I can enjoy weight management and disease prevention.
(1) Strongly Disagree (2) Disagree (3) Neutral (4) Agree (5) Strongly Agree

As you reflect on your self-assessment, celebrate your achievements and acknowledge areas for personal growth. High ratings in body appreciation and cutting out sugar signify a positive relationship with yourself and a commitment to reducing potential health risks. Similarly, crowding out highly processed foods demonstrates a dedication to nourishing your body with wholesome options, fostering overall weight management and mental health.

A high rating in time-restricted eating practices aligns with metabolic health, emphasizing the importance of optimal digestion and autophagy and lowered insulin levels. Prioritizing sleep and aligning with your circadian rhythm is crucial for hormonal balance and overall health. Recognizing and responding to physical rather than emotional hunger showcases mindfulness, contributing to a healthy relationship with food.

View those areas with lower ratings as opportunities for personal adjustments. Identify actionable steps to enhance these aspects of your lifestyle, supporting your transformation toward sustainable metabolic health and overall well-being. Your journey is dynamic, and these self-reflections provide a roadmap for continuous growth and positive lifestyle changes.

Notes _____
_____
_____

Ready, Set, Goal!
Muscle-centric Diet

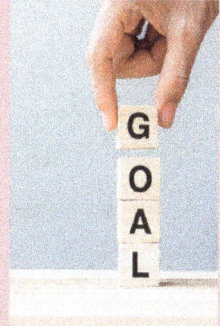

Page 11

You will both have a goal sheet that will require daily reflection and a record of your experience surrounding a muscle-building mindset. Keep the following information in mind when meeting these goals.

You will be asked to track your daily "muscle-centric diet." Here is why:

Prioritizing a muscle-centric diet through protein intake and exercise is crucial for optimal health. Protein is essential for muscle protein synthesis, a process vital for muscle growth and repair. Scientific studies, such as those in the Journal of the International Society of Sports Nutrition, emphasize the importance of protein in maximizing muscle protein synthesis. Combined with targeted exercise, this approach supports muscle development, contributes to fewer cravings, and leads to metabolic health, overall strength, improved body composition, and disease prevention.

HELPFUL Hints

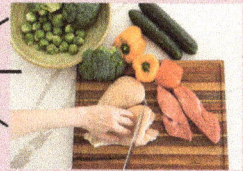

- Each meal should include 30-40 grams of protein
- Optimum levels are 1 gram/ideal body weight daily
- Prioritize quality protein with rich amino acids
- Strength training targeting various muscle groups
- Hydrate to support nutrient transport to muscle
- Adequate rest to allow muscle recovery
- Ensure nutrient-dense foods and protein
- Balance your protein with quality complex carbs
- Eat good quality fat and avoid processed seed oils
- Gradually increase the intensity of workouts
- Establish a consistent routine
- Tune in to your body signals and make adjustments

Notes _____

_____

_____

Ready, Set, Goal!

Muscle-centric Exercise

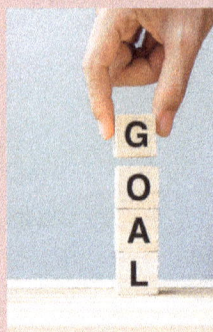

Page 12

As you support each other in making choices that support a muscle-centric lifestyle, stay supportive and encourage opportunities to make optimal daily choices. Learning about the benefits of having healthy skeletal muscle and what is required to attain it is key. This is an important realization as your mindset shifts in the right direction. Pay attention to the world around you and notice you will be set apart from the normal everyday choices of the average person.

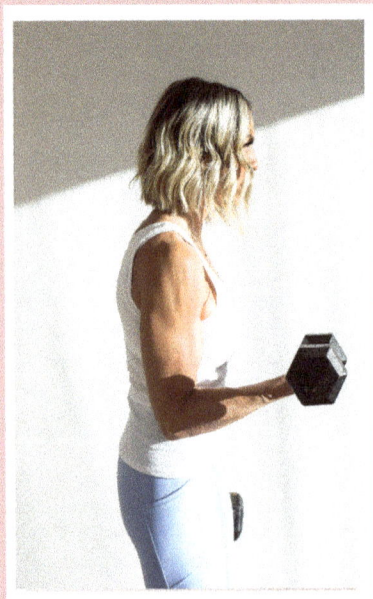

You will be asked to track "muscle-centric exercise." Here is why:

Muscle-centric exercise involves targeted resistance training to stimulate muscle fibers, promoting hypertrophy and strength gains. During resistance training, muscle contraction creates micro-tears in muscle fibers, triggering repair and growth through muscle protein synthesis. Over time, this adaptive process enhances muscle size, strength, and metabolic efficiency. Scientific studies, such as those in the Journal of Strength and Conditioning Research, affirm that structured resistance training positively impacts overall muscle health and contributes to improved metabolic health. Although some may not feel ready for resistance training, other options like walking or yoga still support a muscle-centric lifestyle. Whatever exercise you will sustain is the best exercise!

Notes _____

_____

_____

Ready, Set, Goal!

For Mom

Identifying
your progress
as it leads to a healthy
muscle–centric lifestyle

You can use a tracker like MyFitnessPal, or research the protein grams you are eating. Please write them down daily, and notice your satiety levels rise and your cravings lessen.

Track your type of exercise or rest each day. As you choose one or the other, be intentional as you understand the importance of both when supporting a muscle-centric lifestyle

Daily grams total	Circle one	Exercise	Write down exercise type or rest day
1. _____	Satisfied / Hungry	1. Yes__ No__	_____
2. _____	Satisfied / Hungry	2. Yes__ No__	_____
3. _____	Satisfied / Hungry	3. Yes__ No__	_____
4. _____	Satisfied / Hungry	4. Yes__ No__	_____
5. _____	Satisfied / Hungry	5. Yes__ No__	_____
6. _____	Satisfied / Hungry	6. Yes__ No__	_____
7. _____	Satisfied / Hungry	7. Yes__ No__	_____
8. _____	Satisfied / Hungry	8. Yes__ No__	_____
9. _____	Satisfied / Hungry	9. Yes__ No__	_____
10. _____	Satisfied / Hungry	10. Yes__ No__	_____
11. _____	Satisfied / Hungry	11. Yes__ No__	_____
12. _____	Satisfied / Hungry	12. Yes__ No__	_____
13. _____	Satisfied / Hungry	13. Yes__ No__	_____
14. _____	Satisfied / Hungry	14. Yes__ No__	_____

Notes _____

_____

_____

Ready, Set, Goal!

Page 14   (For Daughter)

Identifying
your progress
as it leads to a healthy
muscle-centric lifestyle

You can use a tracker like MyFitnessPal, or research the protein grams you are eating. Please write them down daily, and notice your satiety levels rise and your cravings lessen.

Track your type of exercise or rest each day. As you choose one or the other, be intentional as you understand the importance of both when supporting a muscle-centric lifestyle

Daily grams total	Circle one	Exercise	Write down exercise type or rest day
1. _____	Satisfied / Hungry	1. Yes__ No__	_____
2. _____	Satisfied / Hungry	2. Yes__ No__	_____
3. _____	Satisfied / Hungry	3. Yes__ No__	_____
4. _____	Satisfied / Hungry	4. Yes__ No__	_____
5. _____	Satisfied / Hungry	5. Yes__ No__	_____
6. _____	Satisfied / Hungry	6. Yes__ No__	_____
7. _____	Satisfied / Hungry	7. Yes__ No__	_____
8. _____	Satisfied / Hungry	8. Yes__ No__	_____
9. _____	Satisfied / Hungry	9. Yes__ No__	_____
10. _____	Satisfied / Hungry	10. Yes__ No__	_____
11. _____	Satisfied / Hungry	11. Yes__ No__	_____
12. _____	Satisfied / Hungry	12. Yes__ No__	_____
13. _____	Satisfied / Hungry	13. Yes__ No__	_____
14. _____	Satisfied / Hungry	14. Yes__ No__	_____

Notes _____

_____

Support & Report

To be done on Day 14:

It's time for show and tell.
Review and plan your future health!

Page 15

Accountability CTA (Call to Action)

This is a time for celebration, reflection, and planning! Congratulations on completing all six modules! This marks a significant milestone in your journey toward a health-driven lifestyle. Take this moment to celebrate your positive changes over the past three months. Your commitment to body acceptance, body recomposition, insulin sensitivity, disease prevention, and sustainable weight loss reflects a profound dedication to your future health. Reflect on the valuable health strategies you have learned – tools that will guide you toward a future of sustainable health. Your newfound knowledge in circadian health, emotional hunger deciphering, and a muscle-centric lifestyle sets the foundation for lifelong health. Continue supporting each other and sharing these transformative tools with your family and friends as you progress. As you set a new standard of health to those around you, encourage them by setting the bar high with your example. As you practice your health standards daily, you will encourage others to modify their standards instead of being tempted to fall into old practices. You have the knowledge – now practice the principles! This is not an end but a beginning. Your journey toward optimal health is well worth celebrating, reflecting upon, and planning for the vibrant future ahead.

It is now time to reflect and plan. What did you find most challenging? Was there anything that surprised you? What is the most valuable thing you learned in all 6 Modules? What is something you wish you had done differently? What are you most proud of? What is something you foresee getting in the way of your future health? How will you prepare and avoid this roadblock? Envision your future self and write down what you will do to achieve that. Get ready – your health journey has its foundation; now, build your healthy future! Congratulations on completing your three-month course!

Notes _____

_____

_____

BOOK SUMMARY

Healthy Echoes is more than a weight loss program. It is a life-changing experience designed to inspire a positive view of body image and a healthier relationship with food, nurturing a legacy of self-confidence and well-being for both mothers and daughters. Learn about preventing PCOS, diabetes, and the role of muscle in insulin resistance, and sustainable weight management. I am excited to present this empowering journey toward healthier, happier relationships with your bodies, your food, and each other.

This educational workbook will take you through six modules. Each Module includes progressive steps toward optimal health and weight management. You will gain knowledge on the following topics:

Body image and nutrition: How eating well is the first act of love for your body. Modeling behavior and how we pick up on a healthy or destructive mind-set. Eliminating sugar and tools to "crowd it out." How nutrition brings confidence. In this Module, we will delve into the science behind the mother-daughter relationship and its role in shaping our perception of our bodies. We will also explore the importance of healthy eating, and crowding out sugar. Most importantly, we will approach the benefits of embracing and appreciating our bodies.

Whole foods and swap outs: How to read labels and combat insulin resistance. Understand cravings and leveraging nutrients while prioritizing protein & healthy fats. How transitioning to whole foods positively impacts our hormonal balance, aiding in weight management and easing symptoms of depression and anxiety. Prioritizing protein and whole foods help to combat various health concerns while providing sustainable energy and controlling cravings. When our nutritional needs are met, our body stops the search for nutrients, resulting in diminished cravings and satiety (feeling satisfied).

Rest and digest: A metabolic reset. Teach your body to use fat as fuel as you learn the benefits of lowering insulin levels and how it pertains to disease prevention & metabolic health. Shifting from sugar burning to fat burning is crucial for sustained energy, improved body composition, and disease prevention. Insulin resistance, a key factor in obesity and diseases, is addressed through time-restricted eating or intermittent fasting. By embracing this method, your bodies will become more insulin-sensitive, promoting efficient energy utilization and reducing the risk of health issues. Together, you will cultivate habits that foster well-being and metabolic resilience for a sustainable lifestyle.

Sleep and circadian health: Aligning lifestyle with the body's natural daily rhythm for optimal health. Understanding Circadian Rhythms and how to create a circadian-friendly lifestyle. This includes managing light exposure and tailoring daily habits Synchronized circadian cycles contribute to improved mood, immune function, and overall well-being. Learn how sleep disrupts hormone and hunger levels. Poor sleep leads to higher glucose and insulin levels which make it harder to manage weight, over consumption of food and cravings. Discovering and respecting your body's natural rhythm fosters lasting vitality, resilience, and a deeper connection to the innate balance of life. Together, you will learn to embrace circadian health for a harmonious approach to your overall health and well-being.

Emotional vs. physical hunger: Learning to establish the difference to optimize nutrition, a healthy mindset, and body. How to recognizing physical hunger and understand emotional hunger triggers by learning mindful eating practices and healthy coping mechanisms. Understanding the distinctions between emotional, mental, and physical hunger is pivotal for optimal nutrition and overall well-being. Recognizing the unique cues of each hunger type enables you to make mindful dietary choices, fostering awareness of genuine nutritional needs. You can avoid impulsive or stress-induced eating by differentiating emotional cravings from physiological requirements. This heightened awareness contributes to healthier eating habits, supporting weight management and a balanced lifestyle. Emphasizing this approach empowers you to nourish your body and emotional and mental well-being, cultivating a sustainable foundation for lifelong health and vitality.

Metabolism and muscle health: Metabolic healing by supporting a muscle-centric lifestyle. Explore a muscle-centric lifestyle and understand a muscle-centric diet while learning the role of muscle-centric exercise and incorporate a mindset for metabolic health. Living a muscle-centric lifestyle is a powerful catalyst for metabolic health. A diet rich in protein and nutrients fuels the body's metabolic engine, supporting efficient calorie burning. Incorporating resistance training builds and maintains lean muscle mass, boosting metabolism and insulin sensitivity. The mindset completes the triad, fostering a holistic approach to well-being. By synergizing a nutrient-dense diet, purposeful exercise, and a positive mindset, individuals unlock sustained metabolic health, weight management, and well-being.

As all six modules come together, you learn the magic of living a muscle-centric lifestyle and the profound health benefits it offers your mother-daughter team. Prioritizing a protein-forward diet and clean, nutrient-rich foods supports metabolic health, promoting sustained energy and weight. Engaging in exercise that stimulates healthy muscle growth not only enhances strength but also aids in disease prevention, fosters metabolic freedom, and contributes to overall weight management. This approach promotes a strong foundation for sustainable, long-term health, weight-loss, fat-loss, regaining insulin sensitivity and creating habits that contribute to a healthy sustainable lifestyle.

This isn't a quick-fix diet. This education workbook offers you and your daughter the knowledge you need to lead the healthiest, most active life possible as you give your body what it needs to thrive and prevent metabolic disease.

---

www.ingramcontent.com/pod-product-compliance
Lightning Source LLC
Chambersburg PA
CBHW052025030426
42335CB00026B/3277